Cerebral Circulation - Updates on Models, Diagnostics and Treatments of Related Diseases

Edited by Alba Scerrati, Luca Ricciardi and Flavia Dones

Published in London, United Kingdom

Cerebral Circulation - Updates on Models, Diagnostics and Treatments of Related Diseases
http://dx.doi.org/10.5772/intechopen.98169
Edited by Alba Scerrati, Luca Ricciardi and Flavia Dones

Contributors
Prasanna Venkatesh Ramesh, Shruthy Vaishali Ramesh, Prajnya Ray, Aji K, Tensingh Joshua, Anugraha Balamurugan, Meena Kumari Ramesh, Ramesh Rajasekaran, Paul K. Thibault, Teemu Myllylä, Sadegh Moradi, Hany Ferdinando, Aleksandra Zienkiewicz, Mariella Särestöniemi, Alba Scerrati, Giorgio Mantovani

First published in London, United Kingdom, 2022 by IntechOpen
IntechOpen is the global imprint of INTECHOPEN LIMITED, registered in England and Wales, registration number: 11086078, 5 Princes Gate Court, London, SW7 2QJ, United Kingdom

British Library Cataloguing-in-Publication Data
A catalogue record for this book is available from the British Library

Additional hard and PDF copies can be obtained from orders@intechopen.com

Cerebral Circulation - Updates on Models, Diagnostics and Treatments of Related Diseases
Edited by Alba Scerrati, Luca Ricciardi and Flavia Dones
p. cm.
Print ISBN 978-1-80355-360-3
Online ISBN 978-1-80355-361-0
eBook (PDF) ISBN 978-1-80355-362-7

Meet the editors

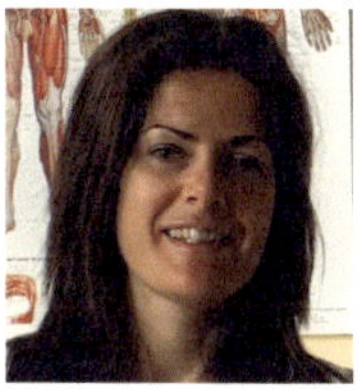

Dr. Alba Scerrati is an Assistant Professor of Neurosurgery, at the University of Ferrara, Italy, and a neurosurgeon at the University Hospital of Ferrara. She graduated from medical school in 2010 and completed her residency in neurosurgery at the Catholic University of Rome, Policlinico Gemelli. Her main scientific interests are skull base surgery and neurovascular surgery. She is working on the development of 3D printing techniques for neurovascular surgery training and simulation. She has participated in different clinical studies on cerebrovascular diseases and CSF dynamics. Dr. Scerrati is the author and co-author of more than eighty indexed publications.

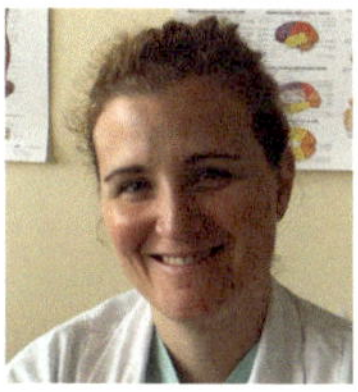

Dr. Flavia Dones graduated from medical school in 2011 and completed her neurosurgical residency in 2017 at the University of Naples "Federico II," Italy. She was previously a neurosurgeon at Niguarda Metropolitan Hospital, Milan, Italy, and in 2019 she moved to Sant'Anna Hospital, Ferrara, Italy, where she is currently working. Dr. Dones' main interests are neurovascular and neuro-oncology surgery. She is the author and co-author of more than twenty indexed publications.

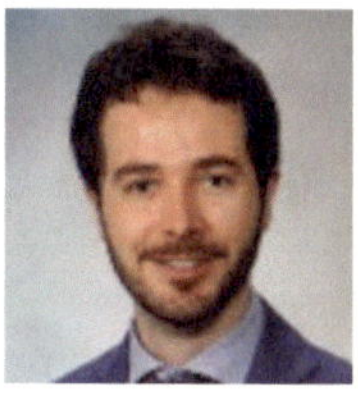

Dr. Ricciardi graduated with degrees in Medicine and Surgery in 2013 and completed his residency in neurosurgery in 2019. In 2017, he completed a fellowship in spinal deformities at the Catholic University of Rome, Italy, and in 2018 he completed a research fellowship at the Mayo Clinic, Jacksonville, Florida, USA. He also completed a four-year training course from the European Association of Neurosurgical Societies and is a fellow of the European. Board of Neurological Surgery (FEBNS). Dr. Ricciardi has authored more than sixty papers published in peer-reviewed international journals. He is a reviewer for more than fifteen scientific journals and has conducted more than eighty certified peer reviews to date. In 2021, Dr. Ricciardi was a guest editor for the *Journal of Neurosurgical Sciences* and an invited editor for *Frontiers in Neurooncology, Life, and Cell*. In 2021, Dr. Ricciardi was nominated as co-chairman and president of the Scientific Committee at SPINE20, the World Congress on Spine Disorders at the G20 conference in Rome, Italy.

Contents

Preface

The cerebrovascular system is characterized by complex anatomy and physiology. Both arteries and veins are responsible for different diseases, some of which are well known (e.g., ischemic and hemorrhagic stroke) and some of which are still being defined (e.g., Eagle jugular syndrome and jugular entrapment, dilated ventricles, intracranial hypertension [JEDI] syndrome).

Diagnostic tests are constantly evolving and 3D augmented reality or measurement of cerebral circulation is giving physicians new information to improve the diagnostic process as well as medical treatments.

The role of the cerebral venous system is being re-discussed considering the new theories about the "glymphatic system" and its function, which seems not to be limited to simple drainage.

This book provides updates on models, diagnosis, and treatment of diseases of the cerebrovascular system.

Alba Scerrati
Department of Translational Medicine - University of Ferrara,
Department of Neurosurgery – University Hospital of Ferrara,
Ferrara, Italy

Luca Ricciardi
Sapienza University of Rome,
Rome, Italy

Flavia Dones
Arcispedale Sant'Anna,
Ferrara, Italy

Section 1

Introduction

Chapter 1

Introductory Chapter: New Models of Cerebral Circulation

Alba Scerrati

1. Introduction

The cerebrovascular system is very complex in its macro and micro-anatomy.

We can anatomically divide the cerebrovascular system into an arterial and a venous compartment.

2. The arteries

Blood flow enters the brain mainly through internal carotid arteries and vertebral arteries. These vessels subsequently create the so-called "Circle of Willis" which is constituted by anterior cerebral artery, middle cerebral artery, anterior choroidal artery, posterior communicating artery, anterior communicating artery, posterior cerebral artery, basilar artery.

Each artery is responsible for the vascularization of a specific cerebral area [1].

Arteries are characterized by anatomical variations and are responsible for several diseases such as aneurysms, arterio-venous malformations (AVMs), restrictions in blood flow that may occur from vessel narrowing (stenosis), clot formation (thrombosis), blockage (embolism), or blood vessel rupture (hemorrhage). These conditions cause a lack of sufficient blood flow to the brain parenchyma and may cause a stroke [2–4].

Standard diagnostic tools for this kind of disease are:

Cerebral Angiography: a catheter for dye injection is usually inserted in the femoral artery and then threaded through the main vessels of the abdomen and chest until reaching the carotid or vertebral artery. Through the use of a fluoroscope after the contrast dye injection, it is possible to have dynamic pictures of cerebral vessels. This is considered the gold standard diagnostic tool for studying cerebral circulation.

CT Angiography: a contrast dye is endo-venous injected, and CT images are subsequently acquired. Visualization of cerebral vessels injected by the contrast dye is possible together with the brain parenchyma. 3D reconstruction of vessels is possible.

Doppler ultrasound: it is a non-invasive, low cost, and rapid diagnostic test able to study the velocity of flow into the cerebral vessel.

Magnetic Resonance Angiogram: it is similar to CT angiography, with the difference that no contrast dye is required, and no ionizing radiations are used.

Indeed, all these diagnostic tools are constantly updated and improved, and this also allows to discover new pathological entities and helps in finding new treatments.

The aim of this book is to help the readers discovering new tools and models for cerebrovascular disease diagnosis and treatment such as augmented reality, 3D animated anatomical models, or new measurements of cerebral circulation.

3. The veins

The veins of the brain have no muscular tissue in their thin walls and possess no valves.

Veins constitute a deep and superficial circulation [1].

The deep parenchymal circulation drains blood from the deep white matter of the cerebral hemisphere, the basal ganglia, and the mesencephalon. Part of this circulation is the Basal Veins of Rosenthal, the internal cerebral veins, and the great cerebral vein (of Galen).

The superficial system comprises dural sinuses and cortical veins.

The superficial cerebral veins can be divided into three collecting systems:

- the mediodorsal group draining into the superior sagittal sinus (SSS) and the straight sinus (SS);
- the lateroventral group draining into the lateral sinus;
- the anterior group draining into the cavernous sinus.

The veins of the posterior fossa are also divided into three groups:

- the superior group which drains into the Galenic system;
- the posterior group which drains into the torcular Herophili and transverse sinuses.
- the anterior group which drains into the petrous sinus.

Venous sinuses are located between two rigid layers of the dura mater.

Venous blood finally leaves the brain through the internal jugular veins or the vertebral system.

If compared to the arteries, veins have always been less considered and studied for cerebrovascular diseases.

For a long time, they have been considered only a drainage system of the brain parenchyma. Indeed, new models and theories have proven a more complex function and their indispensability for maintaining balanced homeostasis of all brain parenchyma [5].

For example the balance of pressure between inflow and outflow in the brain, is mainly maintained thanks to bridging veins.

Moreover, in the past 10 years the idea of a “glymphatic system” has been proposed [6]. This system consists of a sort of “circulation” where cerebro-spinal fluid (CSF) is filtered by the glia limitans and enters the interstitium. It subsequently collects waste products and flushes them to the paravenular space to be discharged. Here, thanks to a balance between venular pressure and paravenular space, it passes into the veins and left the brain. The balance between cerebro-spinal fluid, interstitial fluid, and venous pressure is fundamental to allow this process of “cleaning” the brain parenchyma.

Studies regarding neurodegenerative diseases (such as multiple sclerosis or Alzheimer disease) are being carried on taking into account this new theory [7].

The "occlusive" venous diseases are also becoming more considered and studied.

Cerebral vein thrombosis is a rare cause of stroke (about 0.5–1%), however, it can affect young patients and it is associated with several risk factors, including the SARS-Cov2 infection that since 2019 is burdening the world population [8].

Moreover, new diseases have been associated to vein occlusion, in particular internal jugular vein occlusion.

The JEDI (Jugular Entrapment, Dilated ventricles, intracranial hypertension) syndrome has been described in 2019, consisting of a novel form of high-pressure hydrocephalus that can be successfully treated without a CSF shunt and depending on a bilateral internal jugular vein entrapment at the neck [9].

The Eagle jugular syndrome is characterized by a compression of the internal jugular vein at his passage between the styloid process and the arch of C1. It can be a rare cause of idiopathic intracranial hypertension (IIH) and it can be characterized by headache, tinnitus, insomnia, visual disturbances, or hearing impairment [10, 11].

In this book, a deeper look into new theories and diseases regarding the venous compartment will be discussed.

We hope readers will find interesting hints to improve their daily practice and fields of research.

Author details

Alba Scerrati[1,2]

1 Department of Translational Medicine, University of Ferrara, Ferrara, Italy

2 Department of Neurosurgery, University Hospital of Ferrara, Ferrara, Italy

*Address all correspondence to: a.scerrati@gmail.com

References

[1] Rhoton' s Cranial Anatomy and Surgical Approaches Autori: Rhoton—Congress of Neurological Surgeons (CNS). Oxford University Press

[2] Klötzsch C, Harrer JU. Cerebral aneurysms and arteriovenous malformations. Frontiers of Neurology and Neuroscience. 2006;**21**:171-181. DOI: 10.1159/000092399

[3] Scerrati A, Trevisi G, Sturiale CL, Salomi F, De Bonis P, Saletti A, et al. Radiological outcomes for endovascular treatment of posterior communicating artery aneurysms: A retrospective multicenter study of the occlusion rate. Journal of Integrative Neuroscience. 2021;**20**(4):919-931. DOI: 10.31083/j.jin2004093

[4] Alexandre AM, Sturiale CL, Bartolo A, Romi A, Scerrati A, Flacco ME, et al. Endovascular treatment of cavernous sinus dural arteriovenous fistulas. Institutional series, systematic review and meta-analysis. Clinical Neuroradiology. 2021. DOI: 10.1007/s00062-021-01107-0. [Epub ahead of print]

[5] Scerrati A, De Bonis P, Zamboni P, Dones F, Fontanella M, Cenzato M, et al. A new insight in nonaneurysmal subarachnoid hemorrhage: The potential role of the internal jugular veins. Journal of Neurological Surgery Part A: Central European Neurosurgery. 2021. DOI: 10.1055/s-0041-1733895. [Epub ahead of print]

[6] Li G, Cao Y, Tang X, Huang J, Cai L, Zhou L. The meningeal lymphatic vessels and the glymphatic system: Potential therapeutic targets in neurological disorders. Journal of Cerebral Blood Flow & Metabolism. 2022:271678X221098145. DOI: 10.1177/0271678X221098145. [Epub ahead of print]

[7] Wakamatsu K, Chiba Y, Murakami R, Miyai Y, Matsumoto K, Kamada M, et al. Metabolites and biomarker compounds of neurodegenerative diseases in cerebrospinal fluid. Metabolites. 2022;**12**(4):343. DOI: 10.3390/metabo12040343

[8] Zamboni P, Scerrati A, Sessa F, Pomara C, Mannucci PM. Vaccine-induced immune thrombotic thrombocytopenia with atypical vein thrombosis: Implications for clinical practice. Phlebology. 2022;**37**(3):180-187. DOI: 10.1177/02683555211068948. [Epub 2022 Jan 23]

[9] De Bonis P, Menegatti E, Cavallo MA, Sisini F, Trapella G, Scerrati A, et al. JEDI (jugular entrapment, dilated ventricles, intracranial hypertension) syndrome: A new clinical entity? A case report. Acta Neurochirurgica (Wien). 2019;**161**(7):1367-1370. DOI: 10.1007/s00701-019-03908-2. [Epub 2019 Apr 25]

[10] Zamboni P, Scerrati A, Menegatti E, Galeotti R, Lapparelli M, Traina L, et al. The eagle jugular syndrome. BMC Neurology. 2019;**19**(1):333. DOI: 10.1186/s12883-019-1572-3

[11] Scerrati A, Norri N, Mongardi L, Dones F, Ricciardi L, Trevisi G, et al. Styloidogenic-cervical spondylotic internal jugular venous compression, a vascular disease related to several clinical neurological manifestations: Diagnosis and treatment-a comprehensive literature review. Annals of Translational Medicine. 2021;**9**(8):718. DOI: 10.21037/atm-20-7698

Section 2

Cerebral Arterial Circulation

Chapter 2

Cerebral Arterial Circulation: 3D Augmented Reality Models and 3D Printed Puzzle Models

Prasanna Venkatesh Ramesh, Prajnya Ray, Shruthy Vaishali Ramesh, Aji Kunnath Devadas, Tensingh Joshua, Anugraha Balamurugan, Meena Kumari Ramesh and Ramesh Rajasekaran

Abstract

The field of augmented reality (AR) and three-dimensional (3D) printing are rapidly growing with many new potential applications in medical education and pedagogy. In this chapter, we have used 3D AR and 3D printed models of the cerebral arterial circulatory system, created by us to simplify concept learning. Various cerebral circulation diseases pertaining to ophthalmology can be explained in detail for immersive learning, with the help of various 3D models, for structures such as the circle of Willis, cavernous sinus, various cranial nerves, cerebrum, cerebellum and the eye. These models not only help in cognitive understanding of cerebral circulation diseases but also aid in diagnosing them with better conviction. Ophthalmologists, sometimes being the first responder, have a vigilant role to play with a heightened awareness of these cerebral arterial circulation diseases, which are not only vision-threatening but life-threatening too. This chapter summarizes the construction and holistic application of these 3D ophthalmology-related arterial cerebral circulation models in AR and 3D printing.

Keywords: cerebral circulation, 3D models, augmented reality learning, anatomy redefined, cognitive learning

1. Introduction

Cerebral circulation comprising of both arterial (**Figure 1**) and venous system (**Figure 2**), is a complex three-dimensional (3D) anatomical structure. Various textbooks and chapters have thrown light on the cerebral circulation system with multiple images and various sections of it. Despite that, neophytes may still find it difficult to mentally visualize the complex structures by cognitive 3D mapping. Hence, we have created a 3D model of the cerebral circulatory system and have provided it, both on an augmented reality (AR) platform as well as 3D printed models, to aid in the visual and tactile guide while learning and teaching.

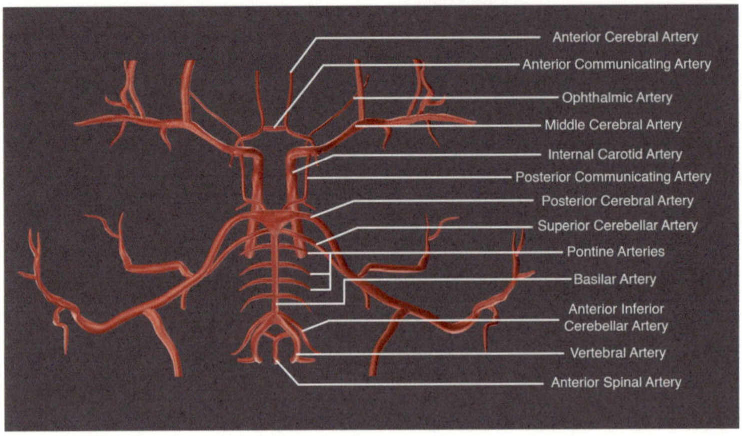

Figure 1.
Image showing the circle of Willis and its parts.

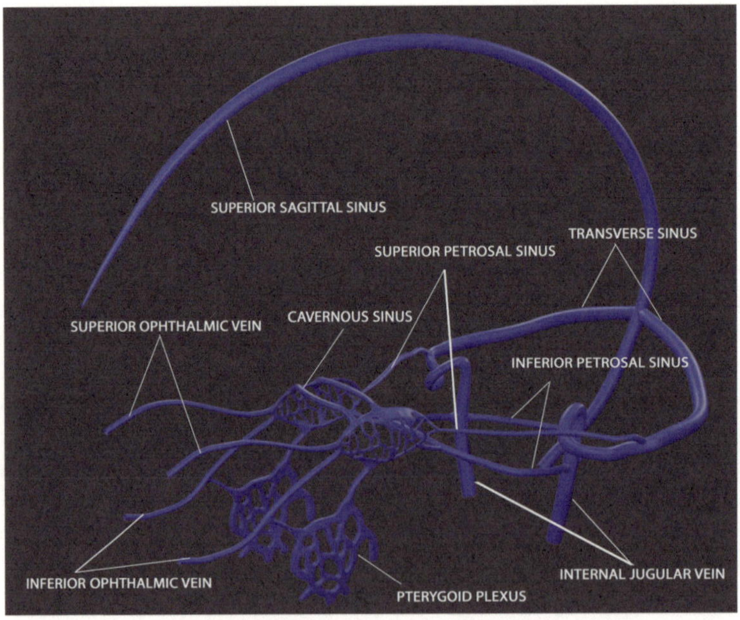

Figure 2.
Image showing the cerebral venous system and its parts.

AR and 3D printed models help in academic-oriented learning of all the cerebral circulation disease conditions and their pathophysiologies [1–4]. We have created 3D models of the cerebral system comprising of various parts such as the cerebral nervous, venous and arterial system along with the brain, brainstem, and eyeball in fine detail (**Figure 3**). By creating these models with meticulous detailing and by incorporating them through AR (**Figures 4–6**), and by 3D printing these models (**Figures 7–9**), understanding of the disease process is made more serene and undemanding with gameful cognitive learning. Also, complex pathways such as the cranial nerve pathways (**Figure 10**) are traced in a three-dimensional manner for facilitating easy cognitive reading.

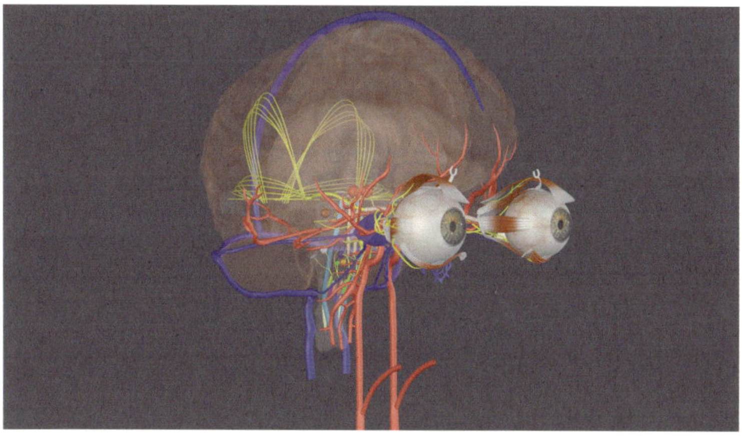

Figure 3.
Image showing the 3D model of the cerebral system comprising of various parts such as the cerebral nervous, venous and arterial system along with the eyeball and its components.

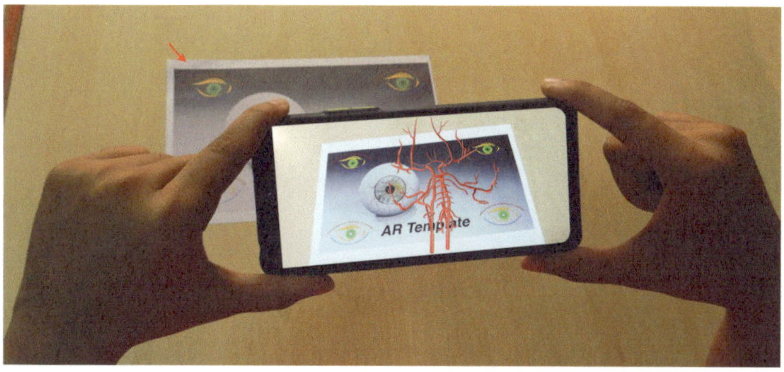

Figure 4.
Image showing the circle of Willis in the mobile screen over the AR template (red arrow).

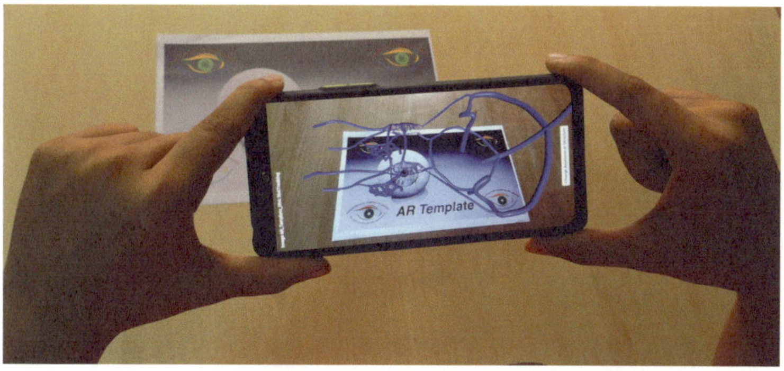

Figure 5.
Image showing the cerebral venous system in the mobile screen over the AR template.

Ophthalmologist may be the first responder for detecting the cerebral pathologies earlier, thus helping in faster diagnosis and aiding in speedy treatment. In this chapter, we have discussed the anatomy of various ophthalmology-related cerebral arterial systems from a neophyte's point of view in detail, with the help of innovative

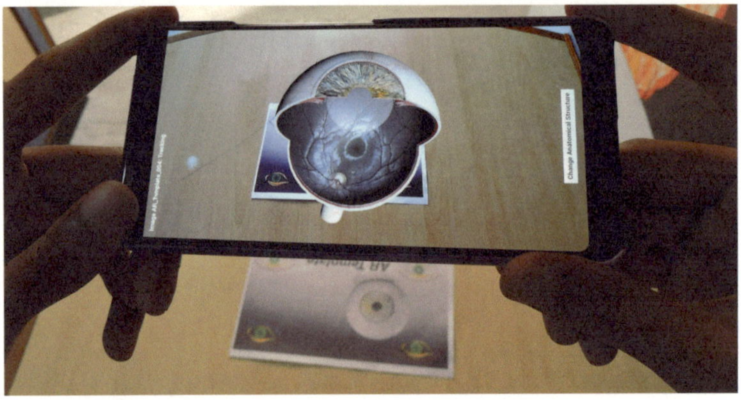

Figure 6.
Image showing the eyeball in the mobile screen over the AR template.

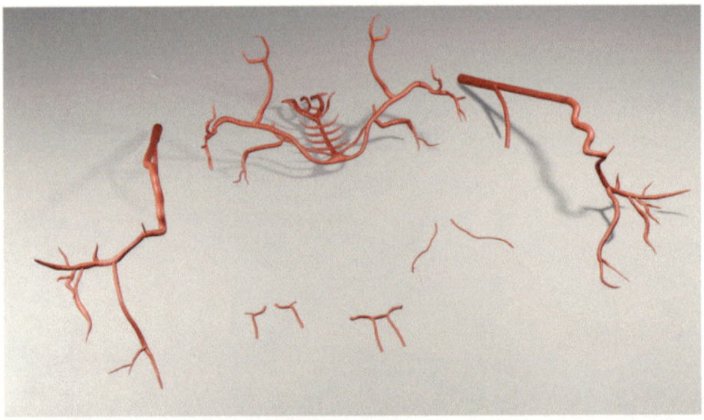

(a)

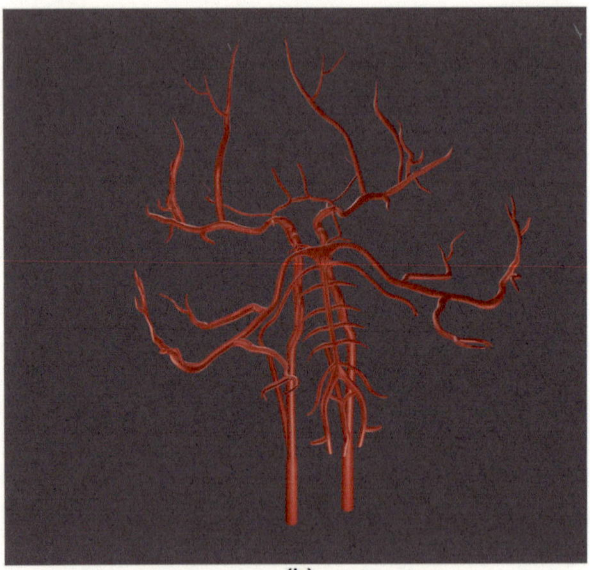

(b)

Figure 7.
(a) Image showing the 3D printed puzzle pieces of the circle of Willis. (b) Image showing the final assembled model of the circle of Willis, after the puzzle pieces are joined together.

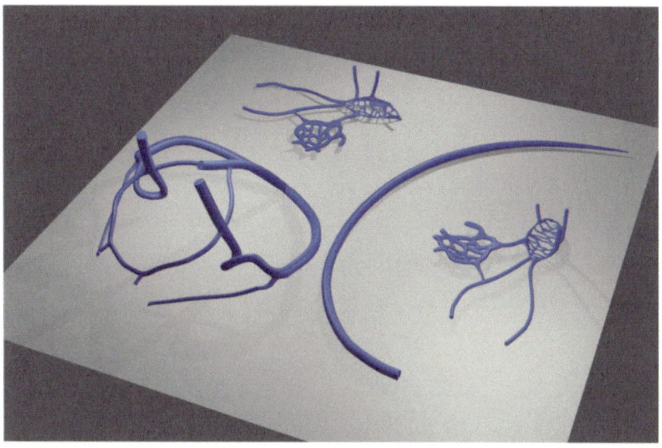

(a)

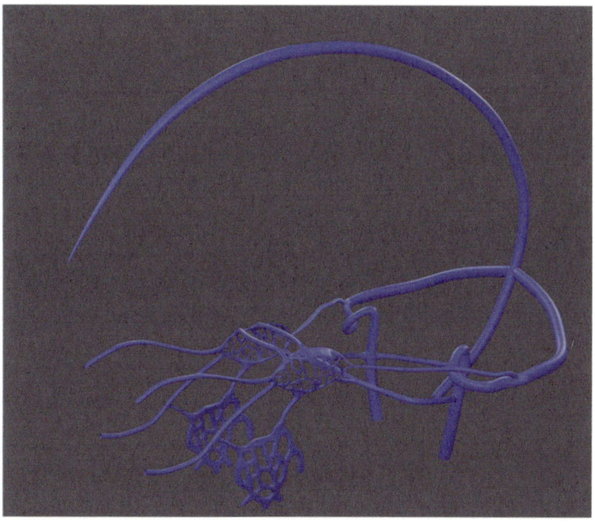

(b)

Figure 8.
(a) Image showing the 3D printed puzzle pieces of the cerebral venous system. (b) Image showing the final assembled model of the cerebral venous system, after the puzzle pieces are joined together.

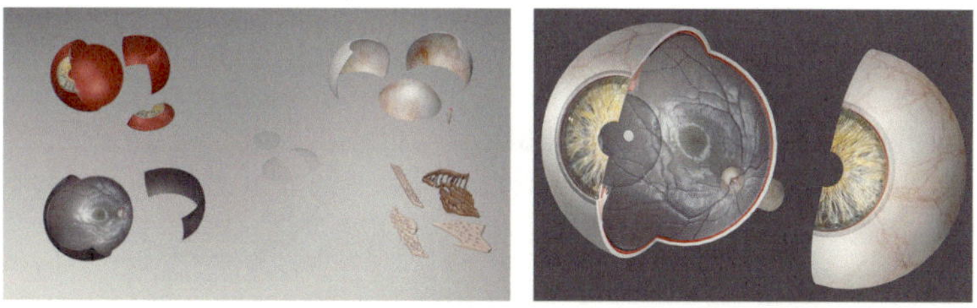

(a) (b)

Figure 9.
(a) Image showing the 3D printed puzzle pieces of the eyeball. (b) Image showing the final assembled model of the eyeball, after the puzzle pieces are joined together.

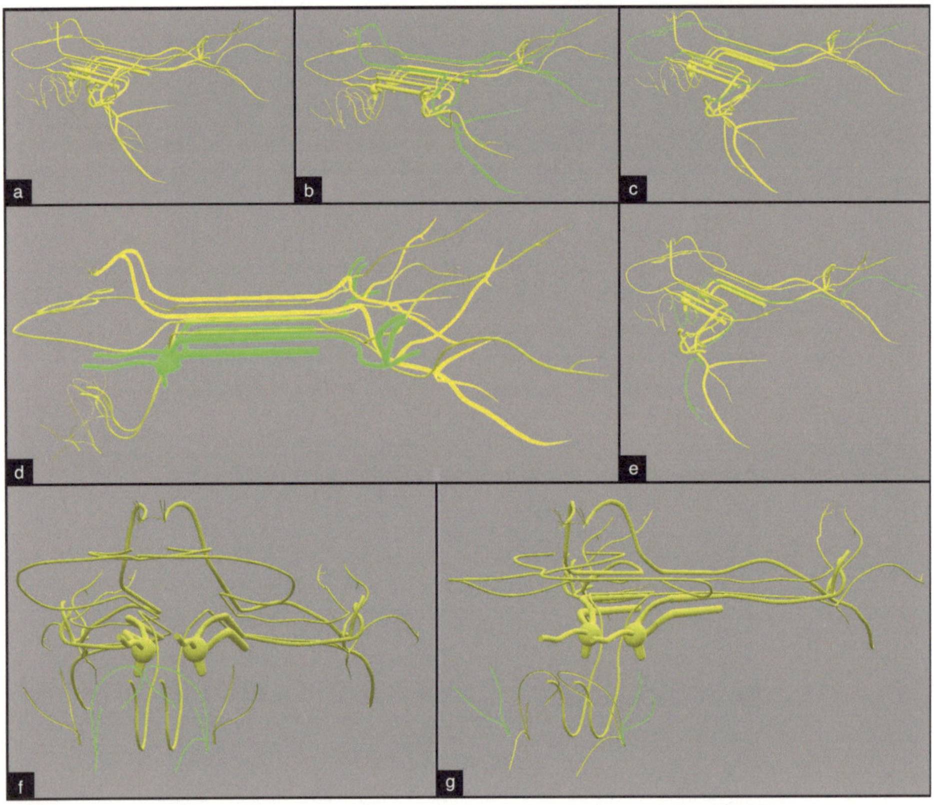

Figure 10.
(a) Image showing the various cranial nervous systems highlighting the (b) 3rd cranial nerve, (c) 4th cranial nerve, (d) 5th cranial nerve, (e) 6th cranial nerve, (f) 7th cranial nerve and (g) 8th cranial nerve respectively in green colour.

3D models and animative video created by us, to simplify the concept learning to aid in timely diagnosis and effective management.

2. Anatomy of the cerebral arterial circulation: Circle of Willis

The circle of Willis (**Figure 1**) is a ring of vessels that provides important colligative communications between the anterior and posterior circulations of the midbrain and hindbrain. The communications are established between the carotid and vertebrobasilar systems in conjunction around the optic chiasma and infundibulum of the pituitary stalk in the suprasellar cistern. It is named after Thomas Willis (1621–1675), an English physician [5]. The circle of Willis plays an important role, as it allows proper blood flow from the arteries to both the anterior and posterior hemispheres of the brain, and defends against ischemia in the incident of vessel disease or damage in one or more areas. In the event of arterial incompetency, it also provides collateral arterial flow to the affected brain regions [6–8].

Vessels comprising the circle of Willis include the following:

- Anterior circulation

- Posterior circulation

Video 1. Animated video depicting the anatomical structures of circle of Willis. Available from (can be viewed at): https://www.youtube.com/watch?v=yCM0Tq9JiFY

2.1 Anterior circulation

When the right and left internal carotid artery (ICA) enter the cranial cavity, each one divides into two main branches:

- Anterior cerebral artery (ACA)
- Middle cerebral artery (MCA)

The ring is formed proximally by a single anterior communicating artery (AComA), which links the bilateral ACAs. Each ICA individually gives off an ophthalmic artery. At the junction between the ACA and the ICA, the lateral continuation of the ICA becomes the MCA.

2.2 Posterior circulation

The posterior communicating artery (PComA) arises from each ACA-ICA junction. The PComA connects the MCA with the posterior cerebral artery (PCA), to form the posteriormost aspect of the circle of Willis. The basilar artery (BA) forms from the fusion of the bilateral PCAs. The BA provides many branches, including the superior cerebellar arteries, pontine arteries, and the anterior inferior cerebellar artery (AICA). From the BA emerges bilateral vertebral artery (VA), which each gives of a posterior inferior cerebellar artery (PICA). The BA artery also contributes to the formation of a single anterior spinal artery [9, 10]. The combination of the AComA and the PComA makes up the circle of Willis, which permits collateral flow between the carotid and vertebrobasilar systems when there is vascular compromise.

2.3 Structures in detail

2.3.1 Internal carotid artery

The ICAs are part of the anterior circulation, which carries major blood supplies to the intracranial contents. There is a total of two ICA; originating from the carotid bifurcation, which runs cephalically through the neck and into the brain. It enters the skull through the carotid canal and reaches the cavernous sinus through the foramen lacerum after passing the parasellar area, and gives off the meningo-hypophyseal trunk that supplies the dura at the back of the cavernous sinus, as well as the oculomotor, trochlear, trigeminal, and abducens cranial nerves. The ICA makes a loop to reverse its direction under the anterior clinoid and the optic nerve at the anterior aspect of the cavernous sinus and passes through the two dural rings. After passing through the second dural ring, it becomes intradural and gives off the ophthalmic artery which is stemming out from the ophthalmic segment (C6) of the ICA. The ophthalmic artery enters into the orbit through the optic canal. It provides numerous collateral branches to supply the optic nerve. The ophthalmic artery's first major daughter branch is the central retinal artery which supplies the retina [11]. The ophthalmic artery provides oxygenated blood to the extraocular muscles, some facial muscles, as well as the intrinsic muscles of the eye [12]. Distal to the origin of the ophthalmic artery, the intradural supraclinoid ICA gives rise to the anterior choroidal artery which supplies blood to the lateral geniculate body (LGB) distally and the optic tract proximally. Anterior choroidal artery anastomoses with the PCA through the PComA. The ICA gives off the ACA and ends as a branch of the MCA [13].

2.3.2 Anterior communicating artery

The AComA connects the two ACAs across the starting point of the longitudinal fissure, organizing the anterior border of the cerebral arterial circle of Willis. Besides forming the conjugation channel between the anterior cerebral arteries, the AComA also contributes to supplying blood to certain parts of the brain via its anteromedial central branches. This artery supplies parts of the optic chiasma and intracranial optic nerves [14].

2.3.3 Anterior cerebral artery

The two ACAs are connected by the AComA. The ACA develops from a primitive anterior division of the ICA that initially supplies oxygenated blood to most midline portions of the frontal lobes, and superior, medial, and parietal lobes. The basal branch arising from the lenticulostriate branch of ACA supplies the posterior aspect of the optic chiasma. The cortical branch and orbitofrontal branch of ACA supply the olfactory cortex, gyrus rectus, and medial orbital gyrus [15].

2.3.4 Posterior communicating artery

The right and left PComAs form the dorsal part of the circle of Willis, at the base. Each PComA links the three cerebral arteries of the same side. Before the terminal bifurcation of the ICA into the ACA and MCA, the PComA connects to the ICA anteriorly. It links with the PCA posteriorly. The PComA supplies the rear part of the optic chiasma and optic tract [16].

2.3.5 Posterior cerebral artery

The left and right PCA is a terminal branch that arises from the bifurcation of the BA. The PCA moves around the cerebral peduncle and supplies the occipital lobe, the inferomedial surface of the temporal lobe, midbrain, thalamus, and choroidal plexus of the third and lateral ventricles after passing above the tentorium. The PCA gives off central branches and cortical branches which supplies the subcortical and cortical structures, respectively. The central branches of PCA include the thalamoperforating artery, thalamogeniculate artery, and posterior choroidal artery. The cortical branches of PCA include the temporal artery, occipital artery, parieto-occipital artery, and calcarine artery [17, 18].

2.3.5.1 Central posterior cerebral artery

The thalamoperforating arteries arise from the P1 segment of PCA and supplies parts of the thalamus, the third ventricles, and the midbrain. The thalamogeniculate artery arises from the P2 segment of PCA and supplies the medial and lateral geniculate bodies and the pulvinar of the thalamus. The medial and lateral posterior choroidal arteries supply the dorsal portion of the thalamus and the choroidal plexus.

2.3.5.2 Cortical posterior cerebral artery

The temporal branches are given off from the P2 segment supply the uncus and the parahippocampal, medial, and lateral occipitotemporal gyri. The occipital branches supply the cuneus, lingual gyrus and posterolateral surface of the occipital lobe. The parieto-occipital artery arises from the P3 segment and supplies the cuneus and precuneus. The calcarine artery supplies the visual cortex, inferior cuneus, and part of the lingual gyrus, which arise indirectly from the occipital artery.

The visual cortex responsible for the contralateral field of vision lies in its domain. The macular part of the visual cortex often receives blood supply from both the PCA and MCA. It describes the "macular sparing" phenomenon in some patients following a PCA infarct.

2.3.6 Basilar artery

The right VA arises from the innominate artery, and the left VA begins as a branch of the proximal subclavian artery. The VA moves through a series of foramina in the lateral aspect of the cervical vertebral processes. After crossing the dura at the foramen magnum, the VA gives rise to the PICA before linking the other VA to form the BA. Along the course of the BA, small branches arise directly to supply parts of the pons and midbrain. The median branches of the BA supply the medial longitudinal fasciculus, paramedian pontine reticular formation (PPRF), and the medially located nuclei of the oculomotor, trochlear, and abducens nerve. The pontine branch of the BA also supplies the front portions of the cranial nerves (particularly the trigeminal nerve) at the point where they exit from the brainstem. Distally, the PICA supplies the inferior cerebellum, which is closely involved in eye movements. The AICA originates from the caudal BA and supplies the pontomedullary junction and the posterior part of the cerebellum. The internal auditory artery which is a large proximal branch of the AICA supplies the facial cranial nerve complex in the subarachnoid space and follows it into the internal auditory canal [19].

3. Creation of the 3D models

3.1 Constructing the cerebral arterial system

The construction of the cerebral arterial system was done in Maya LT software [3, 20]. The reference image was first taken for the cerebral arterial system to e-trace it using the CV curve tool. Tracing of the different arteries was done using the three orthographic views, namely X-axis, Y-axis and Z-axis (**Figure 11**). This results in a cerebral arterial system, which is made up of lines and curves (**Figure 12a**). Next, a circle was extruded along every curve, thereby resulting in a cerebral arterial system made up of tubes (**Figure 12b**); and these tubes were tweaked in a way, that their ends are narrowed and closed (**Figure 12c**).

The other minor appendages and extensions of the circle of Willis were drawn on a plane, followed by deletion of the unnecessary ones and finally the face of the model

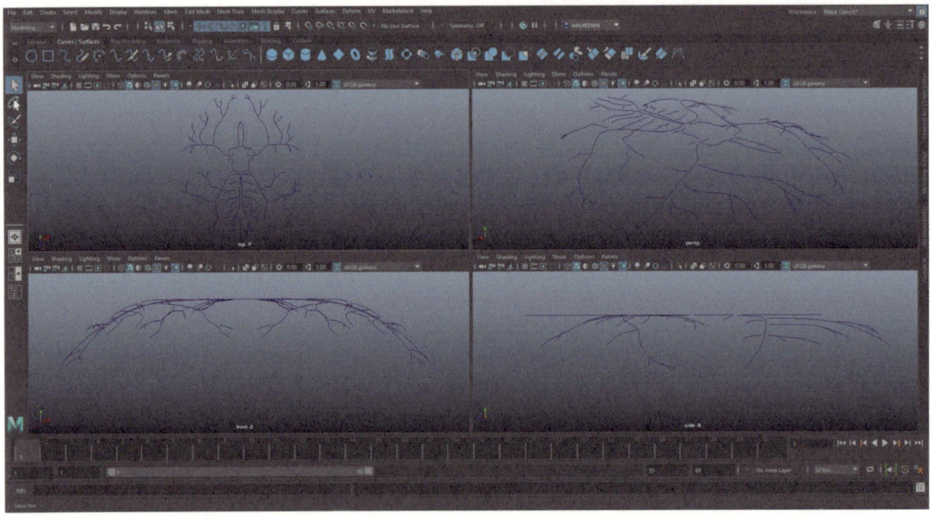

Figure 11.
Image showing the traced cerebral arteries using the CV curve tool in the three different orthographic views namely, X-axis (bottom right), Y-axis (top left), and Z-axis (bottom left). The top right block shows us the default perspective view.

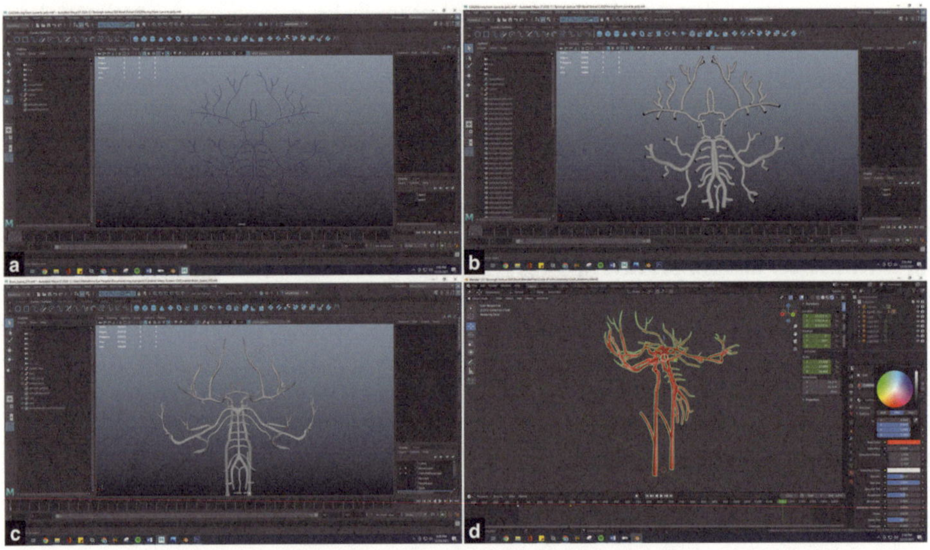

Figure 12.
(a) Image showing the cerebral arterial system made up of lines and curves. (b) Image showing the cerebral arterial system made up of tubes. (c) Image showing the cerebral arterial system with narrowed and closed ends. (d) Image showing the cerebral arterial system with approximated artery colour given from default colour palette.

was extruded. Extrusion is mainly done to provide thickness, so that the thin line will transform into a vessel of appropriate thickness. The face extruded model was then applied to the retopologize function to clean up and smoothen the model. Finally, the circle of Willis was merged with its appendages through edge bridging and offset correction, resulting in the creation of the 'cerebral arterial circulation system' structure.

Similarly, the cerebral venous system, cranial nerves, cerebrum, cerebellum, brain stem (**Figure 3**) and the eyeball with TrueColor confocal images can be created.

3.2 Texturing the cerebral arterial system

The constructed model was given an approximated artery colour from the default colour palette (**Figure 12d**). This step can be done in Maya LT software or Blender software [21]. If Blender software is used, the 3D models have to be first exported from Maya LT software and imported into Blender software.

4. Augmented reality

The 3D models can be successfully launched in AR after UV unwrapping and lighting, followed by coding the models for the AR module in Unreal Engine software for a successful run.

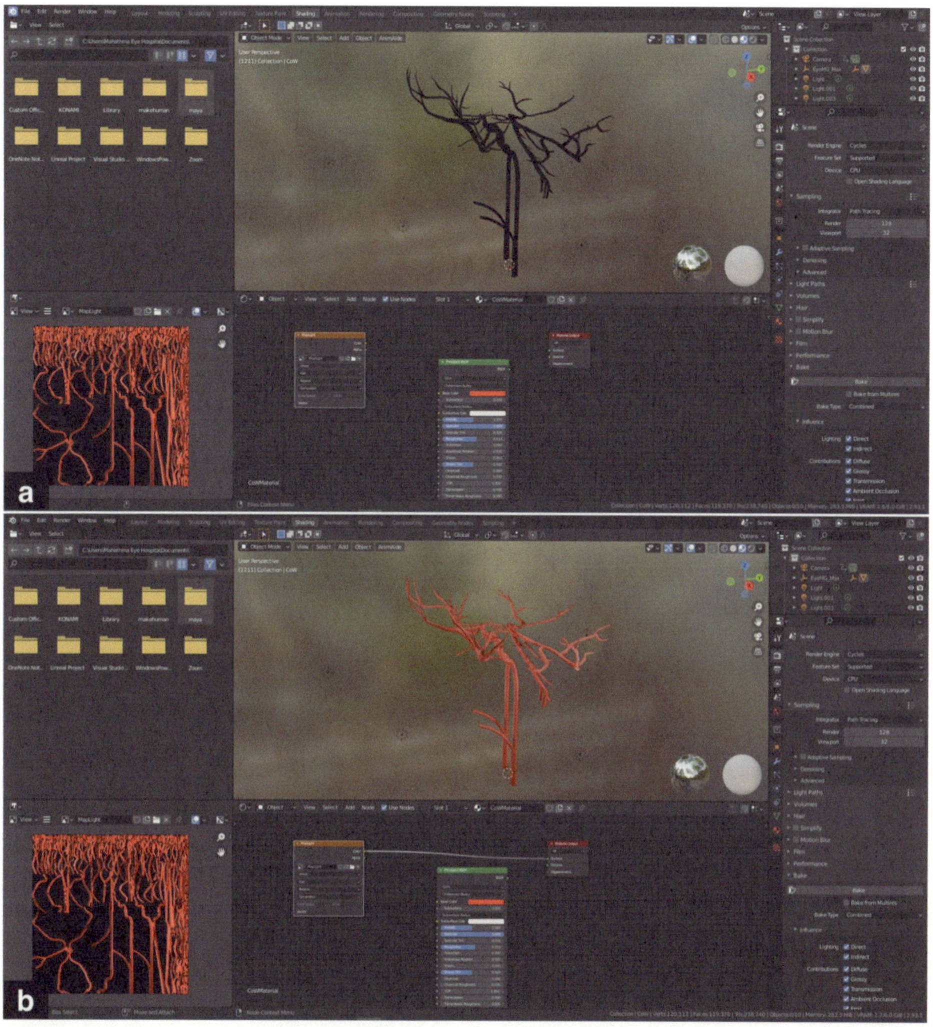

Figure 13.
(a) Image showing the cerebral arterial system is appearing as black due to the absence of lightmap. (b) Image showing the cerebral arterial system is appearing in normal colour due to presence of lightmap.

4.1 UV unwrapping the cerebral arterial system model in Blender software

The 3D models have to be exported from Maya LT software and imported into Blender software for UV unwrapping. UV unwrapping is the process of cutting out a 3D model and placing it on a 2D plane. UV unwrapping is done so that the model can be lit in the absence of scene lights, which is very essential for a successful AR module.

4.2 Lighting the AR scene in Blender software for processing the models in Unreal Engine software

If there is no light in the AR scene, the 3D models inside the Unreal Engine software will appear black (**Figure 13a**). If we add light to the AR scene in the Unreal Engine software, the Android mobile phones will not be able to process it. But, processing the model by the mobile phone is of utmost importance, as the AR module innovated by us needs an Android mobile phone platform to operate. Hence, a lightmap has to be generated and applied to the 3D models to view the models correctly (**Figure 13b**), which cannot be done in Unreal Engine software. Hence, these lightmaps have to be generated in Blender software and then imported into the Unreal Engine.

4.3 Launching the Unreal Engine software for AR

The Unreal Engine is an integrated development environment (IDE) used to develop applications for various platforms [22–24]. The AR application is one such application that was coded in the Unreal Engine software [25]. The 3D models were exported from Blender software after UV unwrapping and imported into the Unreal Engine level file for the initiation of AR. Finally, the app (Eye MG AR) is built from the Unreal Engine for Android devices. The link for the app is given below:

https://play.google.com/store/apps/details?id=com.EyeMG_AR

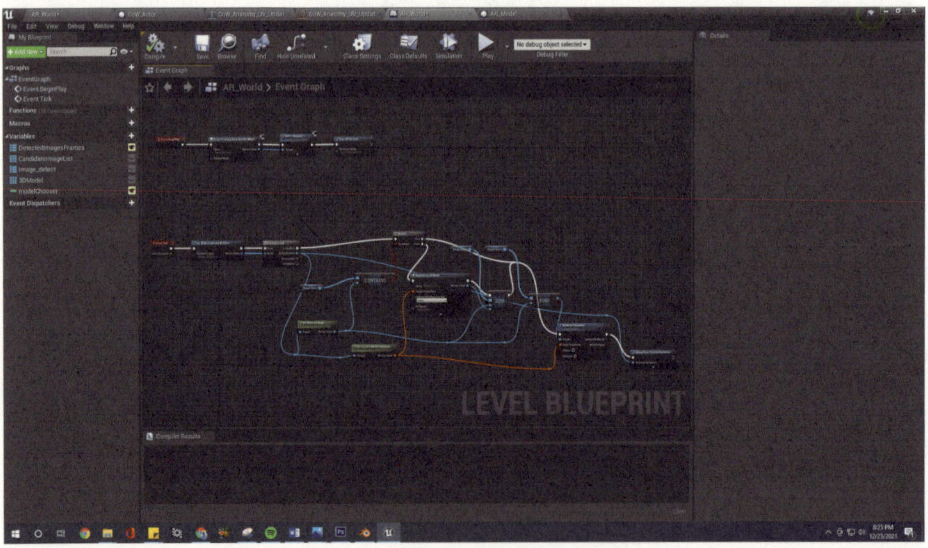

Figure 14.
Image showing the coding/algorithm of the AR module.

4.4 Coding for AR module in Unreal Engine

A dataset array is set up in Unreal Engine software which contains the image of the AR template (**Figure 4**). When the program starts running, all the images in the camera view will be tracked. If any of the tracked images match with the AR template from the data set array, the 3D models will be spawned, with transform values matching the centre of the AR template. If the 3D model is already spawned, then the transform value is updated to the centre of the AR template and will go to the next frame. This is the algorithm for the AR module (**Figure 14**), and it is made to run on a loop at multiple frames per second (FPS) depending on the device.

5. 3D printing anatomy puzzle models

The 3D printing of ophthalmology related models has been proposed first by Ramesh et al. for enhancing learning through the concept of puzzle assembly (**Figures 7-9**) [26]. The concept of puzzle assembly can serve as a comprehensive self-learning tactile tool kit for neophytes [26–31]. 3D printing models can overcome the limitations of the theoretical framework of textbooks used for studying [32–35]. Practical sessions facilitate teaching and 3D printing anatomical puzzle models perfectly augment it cost-effectively.

The software used to create the 3D models was Maya LT. Cura software was used for printing the models in sliced layers. Cura software gives the output in an STL format, which is the standard tessellation language format for 3D printing FabX XL printer was used to print the Circle of Willis model and the eye. FabX Plus printer was used to print cerebral venous system model. Polylactic acid (PLA) material which is a biodegradable plastic, manufactured from corn starch, cassava and sugar cane waste was used for 3D printing all anatomical structures except the retina. For the retina, thermoplastic polyurethane (TPU) material was used for 3D printing.

The 3D models created by us are currently available for free download from the website (mcmi.in).

5.1 Economics

The PLA plastic costs approximately 13.43 USD for 1 kg weight. TPU costs approximately 40.28 USD for 1 kg weight.

The economics involved in 3D printing models is as follows:

- Circle of Willis model costs approximately 6.71 USD for 400 g sample
- Cerebral venous system model costs approximately 6.71 USD for 400 g sample
- Eyeball model costs approximately 26.85 USD for 1 kg sample

5.2 Duration of printing

The duration of printing the 3D models is as follows:

- 10 hours to print: The circle of Willis

- 5 hours to print: The cerebral venous system
- 48 hours to print: The eyeball

6. Conclusions

Cerebral arterial circulation and other allied anatomical structures are best understood with sound knowledge of their complex anatomy. In this chapter, we have simplified the anatomical learning of these complex anatomical structures with 3D AR models (in the free Android app Eye MG AR) and 3D printed models for better concept learning. This cognitive learning module of the cerebral circulation will aid in concept building for neophyte ophthalmologists, neurosurgeons, intensivists, physicians, and paramedics thus aiding in faster diagnosis, speedy treatment and effective rehabilitation.

Acknowledgements

We are grateful to Mr. Pragash Michael Raj (Department of Multimedia), and Mrs. Priyadharshini of Mahathma Eye Hospital Private Limited, Trichy, Tamil Nadu, India for their technical support throughout the making of this chapter and its illustrations. We sincerely express our thanks to Ms. Banasmita Mohanty for her support for the proofreading of this chapter. We are also grateful to Dr. Sabin Malik for his support and help with references for the anatomy of the cerebral models used for animation in this chapter.

Conflict of interest

The authors declare no conflict of interest.

Notes/thanks/other declarations

I (Dr. Prasanna Venkatesh Ramesh) owe a deep sense of gratitude to my daughters (Pranu and Hasanna) and family (in-laws) for all their prayers, support, and encouragement. Above all, I extend my heartfelt gratitude to all the patients who consented to the images which are utilized for this chapter.

I (Dr. Shruthy Vaishali Ramesh) want to thank my partner (Arul) for his constant support and encouragement during the process of creating this chapter.

Declaration of patient consent

In the form, the patient(s) has/have given his/her/their consent for his/her/their images and other clinical information to be reported in the chapter. The patients understand that their names and initials will not be published and due efforts will be made to conceal their identity, but anonymity cannot be guaranteed.

Appendix and nomenclature

3D models were created and used in animations by us in this chapter. This includes the human eyeball with TrueColor confocal fundus image, cranial nervous system, the cerebral venous system, cerebral arterial system (comprising of the circle of Willis), brain stem nuclei, extraocular muscle, meninges etc. These models help in better understanding and can be used in various fields of medicine. We have created models which are related to ophthalmology, which allows us to explain a disease or a condition with its pathophysiology, pathway, clinical features, tests, treatment and prognosis.

These models can be 3D printed, used for augmented reality simulations, used for virtual reality and can also be used for advanced mixed reality with Microsoft HoloLens. 3D models when used for real-time teaching, especially with the help of multimodal fundus images, microscopic structures like the trabecular meshwork, angles, diseases of lens etc., can pave the way for new-age pedagogy. We have created apps using these models like the Eye MG AR (https://play.google.com/store/apps/details?id=com.EyeMG_AR) and Eye MG 3D (https://play.google.com/store/apps/details?id=com.EyeMG_3D) which are based on augmented reality model of the eye and multimodal fundus imaging atlas, respectively. These are available for Android users and are free to download from Google Play Store. An app for iPhone users, named Eye MG Max is currently available in App Store. In this application, eyeball with TrueColor confocal fundus images, and all structures related to ophthalmology are provided with a user-friendly interface. In Eye MG Max, multiple views with transparency for viewing the structures passing through another model, free camera mode, annotated modes, customised zoomed views and videos related to any ophthalmic pathology are provided; thus, providing a 3D atlas at the user's fingertip for comprehensive learning.

Nomenclature

3D	three-dimensional
ACA	anterior cerebral artery
AComA	anterior communicating artery
AICA	anterior inferior cerebral artery
BA	basilar artery
CN	cranial nerve
ECA	external carotid artery
FPS	frames per second
ICA	internal carotid artery
IDE	integrated development environment
LGB	lateral geniculate body
MCA	medial cerebral artery
MLF	medial longitudinal fasciculus
PCA	posterior cerebral artery
PComA	posterior communicating artery
PICA	posterior inferior cerebellar artery
PLA	polylactic acid
PPRF	paramedian pontine reticular formation
TPU	thermoplastic polyurethane
VA	vertebral artery

Author details

Prasanna Venkatesh Ramesh[1*], Prajnya Ray[2], Shruthy Vaishali Ramesh[3], Aji Kunnath Devadas[2], Tensingh Joshua[4], Anugraha Balamurugan[5], Meena Kumari Ramesh[3] and Ramesh Rajasekaran[6]

1 Department of Glaucoma and Research, Mahathma Eye Hospital Private Limited, Trichy, Tamil Nadu, India

2 Department of Optometry and Visual Science, Mahathma Eye Hospital Private Limited, Trichy, Tamil Nadu, India

3 Department of Cataract and Refractive Surgery, Mahathma Eye Hospital Private Limited, Trichy, Tamil Nadu, India

4 Mahathma Centre of Moving Images, Mahathma Eye Hospital Private Limited, Trichy, Tamil Nadu, India

5 Department of Vitreo-Retinal Surgery, Mahathma Eye Hospital Private Limited, Trichy, Tamil Nadu, India

6 Department of Paediatric and Strabismus, Mahathma Eye Hospital Private Limited, Trichy, Tamil Nadu, India

*Address all correspondence to: email2prajann@gmail.com

References

[1] Gopalakrishnan S, Chouhan Suwalal S, Bhaskaran G, Raman R. Use of augmented reality technology for improving visual acuity of individuals with low vision. Indian Journal of Ophthalmology. 2020;**68**:1136-1142

[2] Iskander M, Ogunsola T, Ramachandran R, McGowan R, AlAswad LA. Virtual reality and augmented reality in ophthalmology: A contemporary prospective. Asia-Pacific Journal of Ophthalmology. 2021;**10**:244-252

[3] Karakas AB, Govsa F, Ozer MA, Eraslan C. 3D brain imaging in vascular segmentation of cerebral venous sinuses. Journal of Digital Imaging. 2019;**32**:314-321

[4] Cabrilo I, Bijlenga P, Schaller K. Augmented reality in the surgery of cerebral arteriovenous malformations: Technique assessment and considerations. Acta Neurochirurgica. 2014;**156**:1769-1774

[5] Uston C. NEUROwords Dr. Thomas Willis' famous eponym: The circle of Willis. Journal of the History of the Neurosciences. 2005;**14**(1):16-21

[6] Menshawi K, Mohr JP, Gutierrez J. A functional perspective on the embryology and anatomy of the cerebral blood supply. Journal of Stroke. 2015;**17**(2):144-158

[7] Rosner J, Reddy V, Lui F. Neuroanatomy, Circle of Willis. In: StatPearls [Internet]. Treasure Island, FL: StatPearls Publishing; 2021. Available from: http://www.ncbi.nlm.nih.gov/books/NBK534861/ [Cited: 25 December 2021]

[8] Circle of Willis [Internet]. Kenhub. Available from: https://www.kenhub.com/en/library/anatomy/circle-of-willis [Cited: 25 December 2021]

[9] Prince EA, Ahn SH. Basic vascular neuroanatomy of the brain and spine: What the general interventional radiologist needs to know. Seminars in Interventional Radiology. 2013;**30**(3): 234-239

[10] Robben D, Türetken E, Sunaert S, Thijs V, Wilms G, Fua P, et al. Simultaneous segmentation and anatomical labeling of the cerebral vasculature. Medical Image Analysis. 2016;**32**:201-215

[11] Hendrix P, Griessenauer CJ, Foreman P, Shoja MM, Loukas M, Tubbs RS. Arterial supply of the upper cranial nerves: A comprehensive review. Clinical Anatomy. 2014;**27**(8):1159-1166

[12] Ludwig PE, Aslam S, Czyz CN. Anatomy, Head and Neck, Eye Muscles [Internet]. In: StatPearls. Treasure Island, FL: StatPearls Publishing; 2021. Available from: http://www.ncbi.nlm.nih.gov/books/NBK470534/ [Cited: 15 November 2021]

[13] Internal Carotid Artery [Internet]. Kenhub. Available from: https://www.kenhub.com/en/library/anatomy/internal-carotid-artery [Cited: 25 December 2021]

[14] Gaillard F. Anterior Communicating Artery | Radiology Reference Article | Radiopaedia.org [Internet]. Radiopaedia. Available from: https://radiopaedia.org/articles/anterior-communicating-artery [Cited: 25 December 2021]

[15] Tahir RA, Haider S, Kole M, Griffith B, Marin H. Anterior cerebral artery: Variant anatomy and pathology. Journal of Vascular and Interventional Neurology. 2019;**10**(3):16-22

[16] Posterior Communicating Artery [Internet]. Kenhub. Available from: https://www.kenhub.com/en/library/anatomy/posterior-communicating-artery [Cited: 25 December 2021]

[17] Javed K, Reddy V, Das JM. Neuroanatomy, Posterior Cerebral Arteries. In: StatPearls [Internet]. Treasure Island, FL: StatPearls Publishing; 2021. Available from: http://www.ncbi.nlm.nih.gov/books/NBK538474/ [Cited: 25 December 2021]

[18] Posterior Cerebral Artery [Internet]. Kenhub. Available from: https://www.kenhub.com/en/library/anatomy/posterior-cerebral-artery [Cited: 25 December 2021]

[19] Adigun OO, Reddy V, Sevensma KE. Anatomy, Head and Neck, Basilar Artery. In: StatPearls [Internet]. Treasure Island, FL: StatPearls Publishing; 2021. Available from: http://www.ncbi.nlm.nih.gov/books/NBK459137/ [Cited: 25 December 2021]

[20] Abdul Ghani D, Naim Bin Supian M, Zulhilmi Bin Abdul 'Alim L. The research of 3D modeling between visual & creativity. International Journal of Innovative Technology and Exploring Engineering. 2019;**8**(11S2):180-186

[21] 3D Texturing in Animation; Step by Step Workflow + Techniques & Video [Internet]. Available from: https://dreamfarmstudios.com/blog/getting-to-know-3d-texturing-in-animation-production/ [Cited: 25 December 2021]

[22] Ramesh PV, Aji K, Joshua T, Ramesh SV, Ray P, Raj PM, et al. Immersive photoreal new-age innovative gameful pedagogy for e-ophthalmology with 3D augmented reality. Indian Journal of Ophthalmology. 2022;**70**(1):275-280

[23] Ramesh PV, Aji K, Ray P, et al. Combating anti-glaucoma medication compliance issues among literate urban Indian population—Has this fallen in our blind spot? Journal of Clinical Ophthalmology. 2021;**5**(S5):472-475

[24] Aydındoğan G, Kavaklı K, Şahin A, Artal P, Ürey H. Applications of augmented reality in ophthalmology. Biomedical Optics Express. 2020;**12**:511-538

[25] Eye MG AR—Apps on Google Play [Internet]. Available from: https://play.google.com/store/apps/details?id=com.EyeMG_AR&hl=en&gl=IN [Cited: 26 November 2021]

[26] 3D Printing. In: Wikipedia [Internet]. 2021. Available from: https://en.wikipedia.org/w/index.php?title=3D_printing&oldid=1045923488 [Cited: 5 October 2021]

[27] Sehnonimo. 3D Jigsaw Puzzles and Their Benefits [Internet]. HubPages. Available from: https://discover.hubpages.com/games-hobbies/3D-Puzzle [Cited: 5 October 2021]

[28] Akkara JD, Kuriakose A. The magic of three-dimensional printing in ophthalmology. Kerala Journal of Ophthalmology. 2018;**30**:209-215

[29] Adams JW, Paxton L, Dawes K, Burlak K, Quayle M, McMenamin PG. 3D printed reproductions of orbital dissections: A novel mode of visualising anatomy for trainees in ophthalmology or optometry. The British Journal of Ophthalmology. 2015;**99**(9):1162-1167

[30] Dave TV, Tiple S, Vempati S, Palo M, Ali MJ, Kaliki S, et al. Low-cost three-dimensional printed orbital template-assisted patient-specific implants for the correction of spherical orbital implant migration. Indian Journal of Ophthalmology. 2018;**66**(11):1600-1607

[31] Harrington Z. 7 Spectacular Benefits of Puzzles (Hint: They're Not What You'd Think!) | Melissa & Doug Blog [Internet]. Available from: https://www.melissaanddoug.com/on/demandware.store/Sites-melissaanddoug-Site/en_US/Blog-PostView?postId=7-spectacular-benefits-of-puzzles-hint-theyre-not-what-youd-think [Cited: 5 October 2021]

[32] Sommer AC, Blumenthal EZ. Implementations of 3D printing in ophthalmology. Graefe's Archive for Clinical and Experimental Ophthalmology. 2019;**257**(9):1815-1822

[33] 3-D Printing for Ophthalmic Surgery [Internet]. American Academy of Ophthalmology; 2019. Available from: https://www.aao.org/eyenet/academy-live/detail/3-d-printing-ophthalmic-surgery [Cited: 25 December 2021]

[34] Implications of 3D Printing in Ophthalmology [Internet]. Available from: https://www.longdom.org/proceedings/implications-of-3d-printing-in-ophthalmology-54045.html [Cited: 25 December 2021]

[35] The Application of 3D Printing in Ophthalmology [Internet]. CJEO Journal. 2020. Available from: https://cjeo-journal.org/the-application-of-3d-printing-in-ophthalmology/ [Cited: 25 December 2021]

Chapter 3

Diagnosis and Treatment of Ophthalmology Related Cerebral Arterial Circulation Diseases: A 3D Animated Encyclopedia

Prasanna Venkatesh Ramesh, Shruthy Vaishali Ramesh, Prajnya Ray, Aji Kunnath Devadas, Tensingh Joshua, Anugraha Balamurugan, Meena Kumari Ramesh and Ramesh Rajasekaran

Abstract

Cerebral circulation is the flow of blood through a group of arteries and veins which supply the brain. There are various diseases related to ophthalmology, due to pathologies in the cerebral arterial system. Arteries inside the skull can be blocked by plaque or disease, which in turn triggers a series of events leading to various cranial nerve palsies, visual fields defects, retinal diseases, etc. The highlights of this chapter are the novel three-dimensional (3D) animative videos created by us, to simplify various cerebral arterial circulation diseases and their diagnostic concepts for neophytes. 3D animative videos can aid learning and help in the cognitive concept building of these complex pathologies.

Keywords: cerebral arterial circulation, 3D animations, ophthalmology related diseases, aneurysms, stroke

1. Introduction

Cerebrovascular disease is the 2nd most common cause of death in the world and the 6th most common cause of disability [1, 2]. Cerebrovascular diseases occur primarily during old age. The risk of cerebrovascular disease occurring increases significantly after 65 years of age.

Cerebrovascular conditions include aneurysms, arteriovenous malformations (AVM), cerebral cavernous malformations (CCM), arteriovenous fistula (AVF), carotid-cavernous fistula (CCF), carotid stenosis, transient ischemic attack (TIA), and stroke [3–9]. In this chapter, various cerebral arterial circulation diseases related to ophthalmology are explained in detail using detailed three-dimensional (3D) animative videos.

2. Pathologies

2.1 Anterior communicating artery aneurysms

It can lead to visual field defects and visual deterioration such as bitemporal heteronymous, psychopathology, and frontal lobe pathologies are shown in Video Clip 1 [10].

(Video 1, https://www.youtube.com/watch?v=HoQNbzUTJu0).

2.2 Posterior communicating artery aneurysm

Oculomotor nerves are more prone to damage from posterior communicating artery (PComA) aneurysms. Pathophysiology and clinical features of oculomotor nerve palsy are shown in **Figure 1** and Video Clip 2, respectively [10, 11].

(Video 2, https://www.youtube.com/watch?v=EZ9sQksL_oc).

2.3 Terson's syndrome

Terson's syndrome (TS) is the occurrence of intraocular haemorrhage, manifesting as vitreous, subhyaloid, intraretinal bleeding, or subretinal bleeding, which typically occurs in a setting of traumatic brain injury associated with intracranial haemorrhage [12]. The pathophysiology of TS is shown in **Figure 2**. The clinical features of TS primarily depend on the patient's neurological status and the location of the haemorrhage.

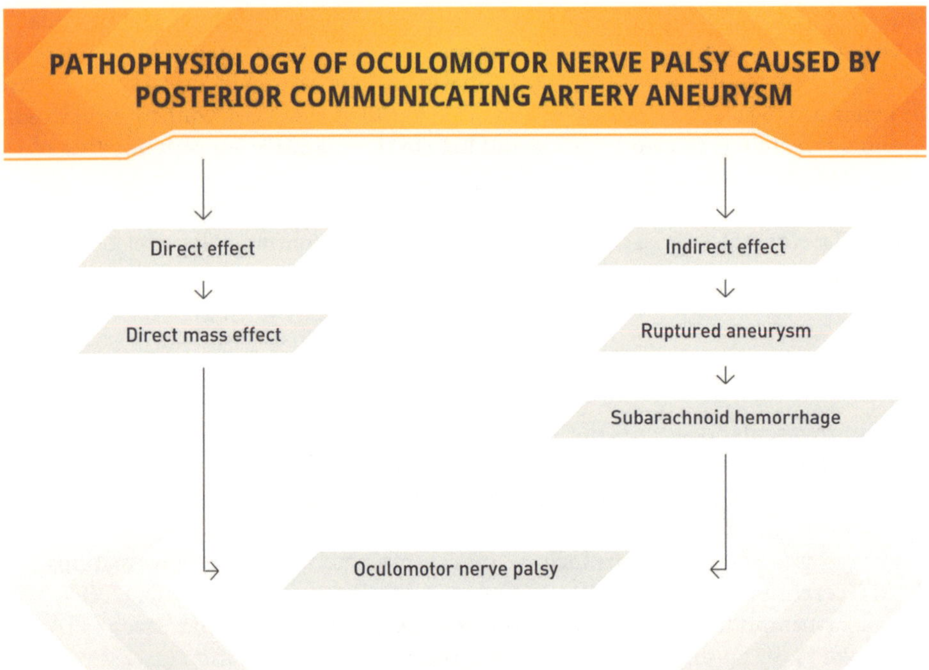

Figure 1.
Pathophysiology of oculomotor nerve palsy caused by posterior communicating artery aneurysm.

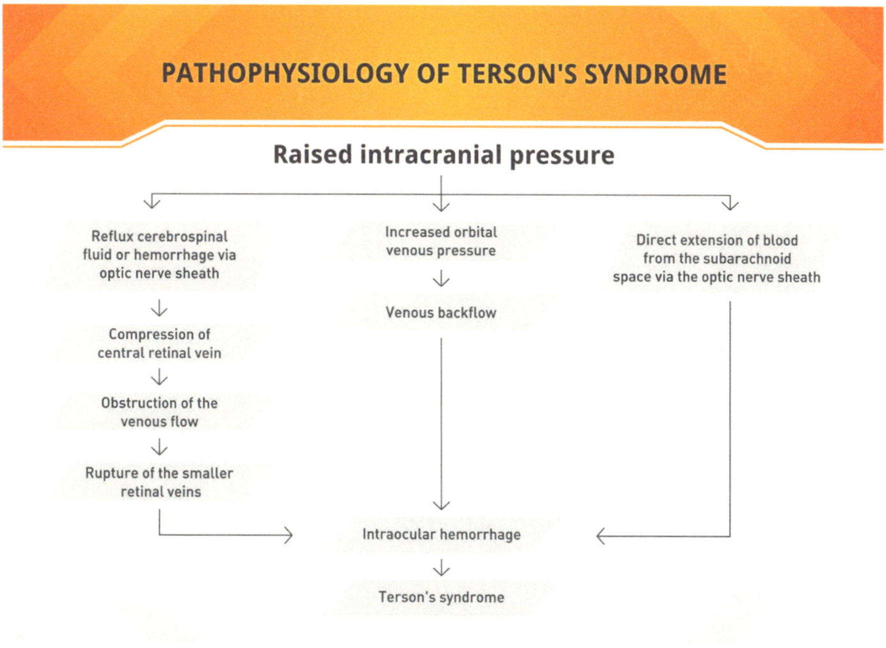

Figure 2.
Pathophysiology of Terson's syndrome due to raised intracranial pressure.

2.4 Posterior inferior cerebellar artery syndrome or lateral medullary syndrome

Lateral medullary syndrome (LMS) occurs due to vascular insult in the lateral part of the medulla oblongata [13]. It was named after a Jewish neurologist, Adolf Wallenberg [14]. The aetiology of LMS is shown in **Figure 3**. The patient presents with clinical features of vertigo, ataxia, nystagmus, oscillopsia, diplopia, dysphagia, nausea, vomiting, headache, impairment of pain and thermal sensation, ipsilateral Horner's syndrome, ipsilateral limb ataxia, dysphonia, hiccups and ipsilateral hyperalgesia. The specific ophthalmic clinical sign for LMS is ipsipulsion.

2.5 Carotid-cavernous fistula

Carotid-cavernous fistula (CCF) occurs due to an abnormal connection between the carotid artery and the cavernous sinus. It can be classified as direct or indirect CCF [15, 16]. Types of CCF are shown in **Figure 4** and Video Clip 3. (Video 3, https://www.youtube.com/watch?v=PYE_NveoIoo).

2.6 Brainstem stroke syndromes

The ocular manifestations that occur in patients with brainstem stroke due to vascular ischemia are shown in **Figure 5**.

2.6.1 Oculomotor nerve palsy

Isolated third nerve palsies are rare; hence it is important to evaluate other cranial nerves and the peripheral nervous system [17]. Clinical features of oculomotor nerve palsy are shown in Video Clip 4.

(Video 4, https://www.youtube.com/watch?v=erN1kQ9-vuk).

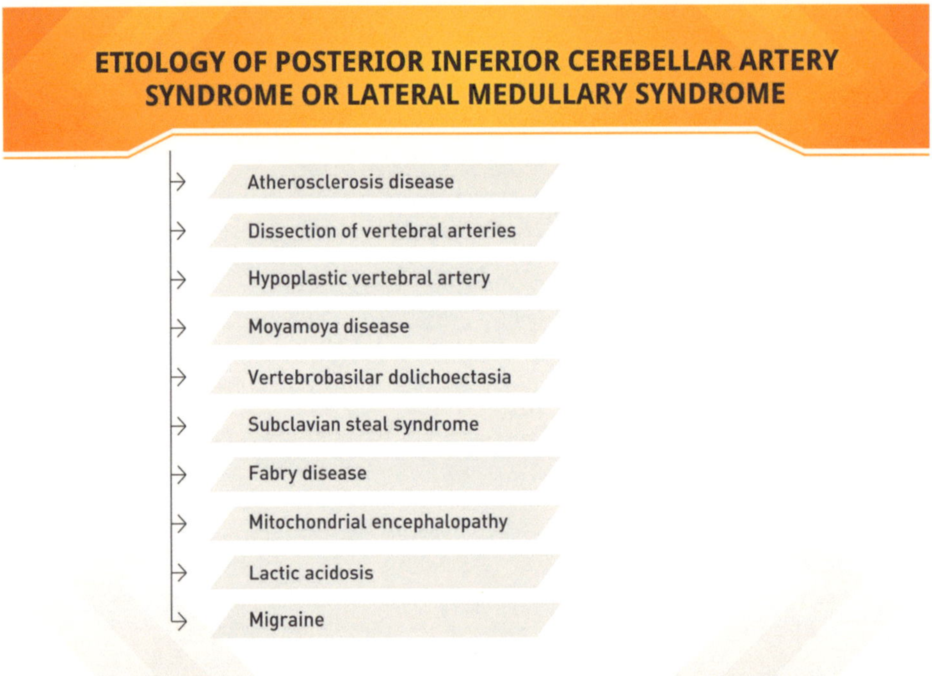

Figure 3.
Aetiology of posterior inferior cerebellar artery syndrome or lateral medullary syndrome.

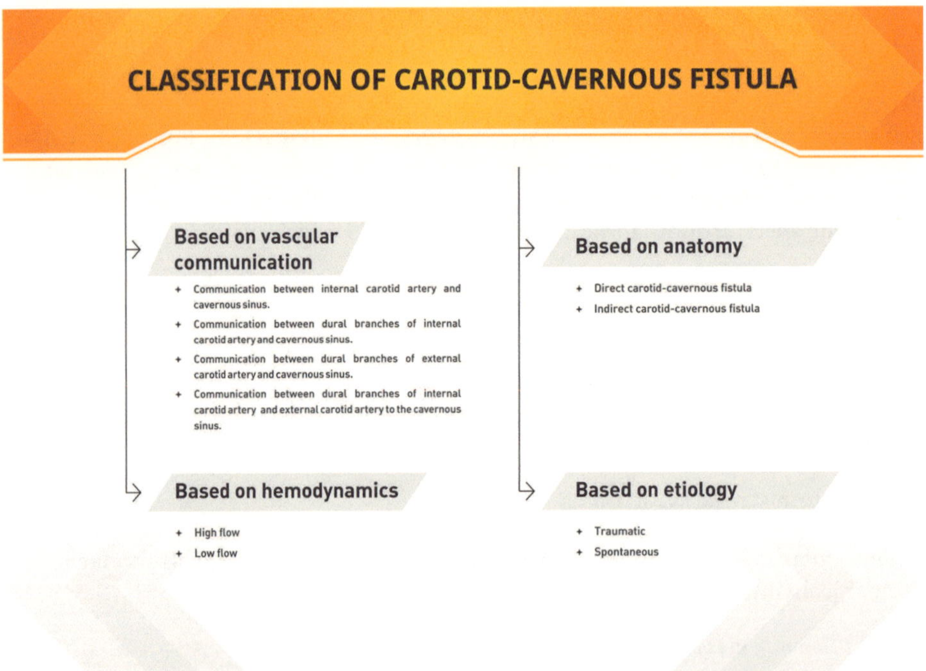

Figure 4.
Classifications of carotid-cavernous fistula.

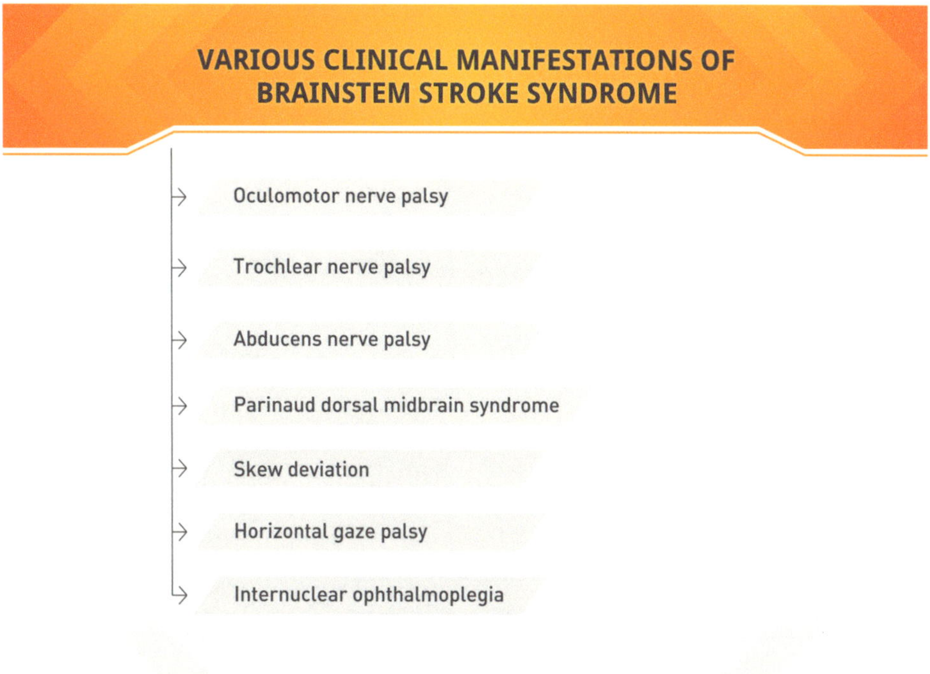

Figure 5.
Various ocular manifestations of the brainstem stroke syndrome.

2.6.2 Trochlear nerve palsy

The patient typically presents with binocular diplopia which is vertical or torsional. Park-Bielschowsky three-step test (**Figure 6**) has been proposed to identify superior oblique palsy in such patients [18]. Clinical features of trochlear nerve palsy are shown in Video Clip 5.

(Video 5, https://www.youtube.com/watch?v=GOYj1EoN3Ss).

2.6.3 Abducens nerve palsy

The patient presents with horizontal diplopia and esotropia, due to unopposed action of the medial rectus. Abduction of the affected side will be restricted. The patient will adapt a compensatory face turn towards the side of paralysed muscle [19, 20]. Clinical features of abducens nerve palsy are shown in Video Clip 6.

(Video 6, https://www.youtube.com/watch?v=Ecuve0RiTZQ).

2.6.4 Parinaud dorsal midbrain syndrome

The clinical triad of parinaud dorsal midbrain syndrome (**Figure 7**) is supranuclear upgaze palsy, convergence retraction nystagmus, and light-near dissociation [21, 22]. Clinical features of parinaud dorsal midbrain syndrome are shown in Video Clip 7.

(Video 7, https://www.youtube.com/watch?v=PF3n6fVEZ3o).

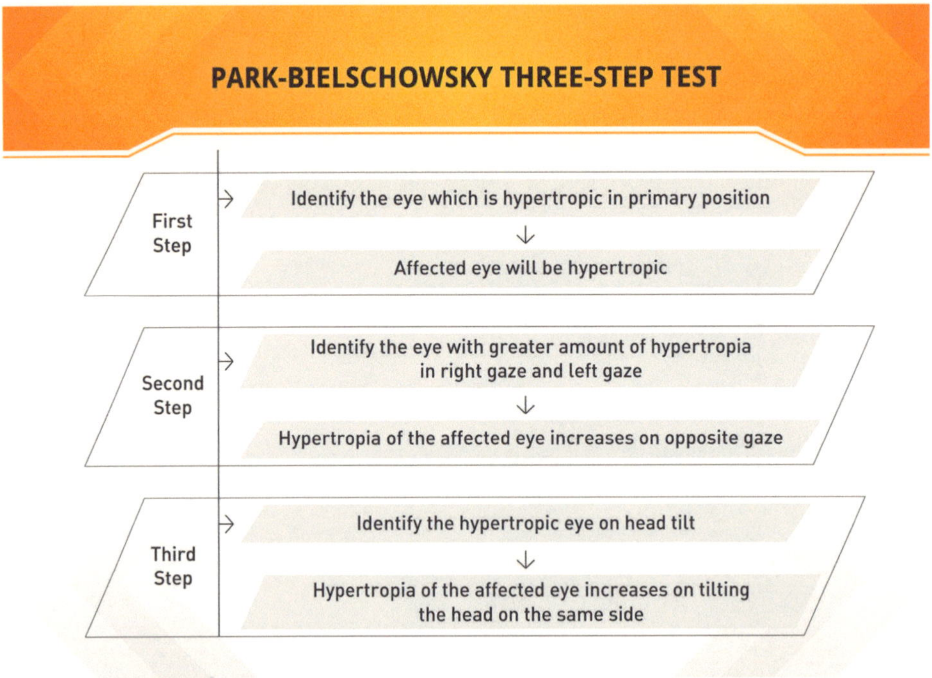

Figure 6.
Park-Bielschowsky three-step test to identify superior oblique palsy.

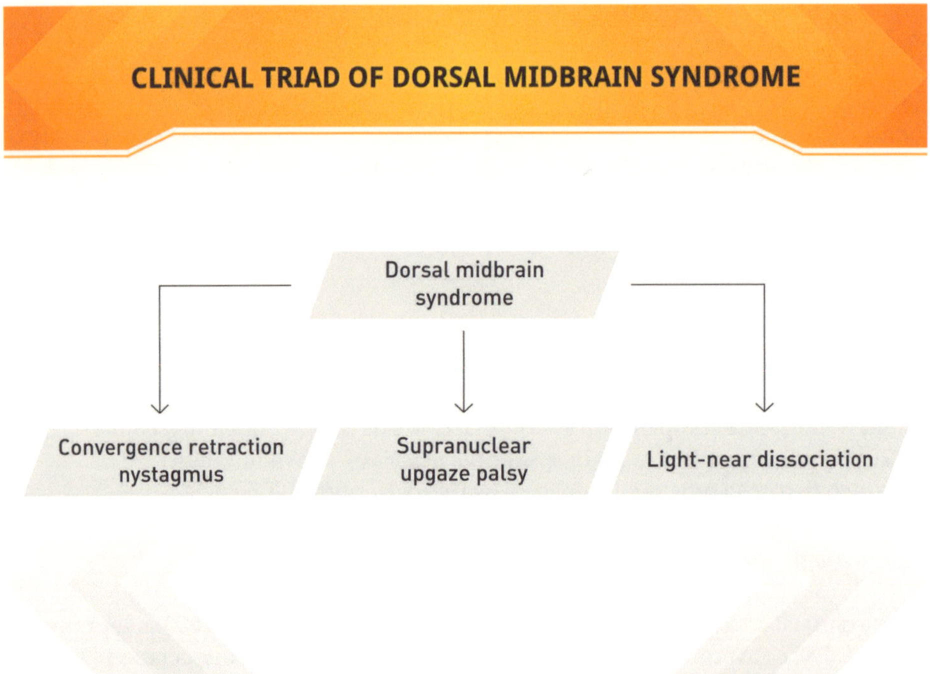

Figure 7.
Clinical triad of dorsal midbrain syndrome.

2.6.5 Skew deviation

It is a supranuclear motility disorder that occurs due to brainstem or cerebellar stroke. The eyes deviate vertically and often present with cyclotorsional disturbances [23]. Clinical features of skew deviation are shown in Video Clip 8.

(Video 8, https://www.youtube.com/watch?v=1GeTQTpozJ4).

2.6.6 Horizontal gaze palsy

Ipsilateral horizontal gaze palsy is caused by a lesion in the horizontal gaze centre of paramedian pontine reticular formation (PPRF), which clinically manifests as an inability to look in the direction of the lesion. Clinical features of horizontal gaze palsy are shown in Video Clip 9.

(Video 9, https://www.youtube.com/watch?v=NQt_-nkcfuA).

2.6.7 Internuclear ophthalmoplegia

Ischemia in the vertebrobasilar system can produce an ischemic internuclear ophthalmoplegia (INO) [24]. In cases of unilateral INO, it clinically manifests as adduction deficit, where defective adduction of the eye will be present on the side of the lesion and nystagmus of the contralateral eye on abduction will be noted [25]. Bilateral INO will lead to defective left adduction and abduction nystagmus of the right eye on the right gaze and defective right adduction and abduction nystagmus of the left eye on the left gaze. Clinical features of internuclear ophthalmoplegia are shown in Video Clip 10.

(Video 10, https://www.youtube.com/watch?v=bQH1wPmN5aE).

2.6.7.1 Wall-eyed bilateral internuclear ophthalmoplegia

Exotropia (XT) need not be present in all cases of bilateral INO. The most common aetiology of wall-eyed bilateral internuclear ophthalmoplegia (WEBINO) is infarction at the level of the midbrain [26].

2.6.7.2 Wall-eyed monocular internuclear ophthalmoplegia

In wall-eyed monocular internuclear ophthalmoplegia (WEMINO), patients will have a unilateral medial longitudinal fasciculus (MLF) lesion with primary position XT [27].

2.6.7.3 One and a half syndrome

The patient will retain only the abduction of the contralateral eye, which will exhibit abduction nystagmus [28]. This condition is termed as one and a half syndrome.

2.6.7.4 Eight and a half syndrome

There is also conjugate horizontal gaze palsy on looking to one side, followed by INO on looking to the opposite side, along with ipsilateral lower motor neuron (LMN) facial weakness [29]. This condition is termed as eight and a half syndrome.

2.6.7.5 Half and half syndrome

There is 'half' of a horizontal gaze palsy plus half of the ipsilateral gaze (abduction deficit from CN VI fascicular palsy) [30]. This condition is termed as half and half syndrome.

2.6.7.6 Posterior INO of Lutz

Lesions interrupting the fibre tracts that connect the pontine centre for conjugate horizontal gaze and the ipsilateral abducens nucleus can cause posterior INO of Lutz [31].

2.7 Chiasmal strokes

Chiasmal strokes typically present as bitemporal hemianopia [32]. In cases of anterior chiasmal strokes, it will produce central scotoma in one eye and temporal field defects in the other eye [33, 34]. Clinical features of chiasmal strokes are shown in Video Clip 11.
(Video 11, https://www.youtube.com/watch?v=mMy2C_AN-Ho).

2.8 Post chiasmal strokes

Clinical features of post chiasmal stroke are shown in Video Clip 11.
(Video 11, https://www.youtube.com/watch?v=mMy2C_AN-Ho).

2.8.1 Optic tract stroke

Lesions usually produce contralateral incongruous homonymous hemianopia along with optic tract syndrome [35].

2.8.2 Lateral geniculate body stroke

In case of extensive lateral geniculate body (LGB) injury, it would produce complete homonymous hemianopia [36, 37].

2.8.3 Optic radiation stroke

Lesions of the anterior optic radiation cause incongruous visual field defects. The field defects become more congruous as it goes more posterior [37].

2.8.4 Temporal lobe stroke

Contralateral homonymous superior quadrantanopia ("pie-in-the-sky" defect), occurs with temporal lobe infarction involving Meyer's Loop, which constitutes the inferior visual fibres [38].

2.8.5 Parietal lobe stroke

Contralateral homonymous inferior quadrantanopia ("pie-on-the-floor" defect) occurs, with additional systemic manifestations depending on the side of the lesion [39, 40].

2.8.6 Occipital lobe stroke

Most occipital lobe lesions are a result of a stroke at the level of the posterior cerebral artery (PCA) and will cause no neurological deficits other than vision loss. Occipital lobe lesions can produce a varied presentation of visual field defects [38].

3. Investigations

- Gold standard modalities for investigating anterior and posterior communicating artery aneurysms are magnetic resonance angiography (MRA), computed tomography angiography (CTA), lumbar puncture (LP), cerebral angiogram and digital subtraction angiography (DSA).

- Regarding Terson's syndrome, if necessary, an ultrasound B-scan imaging of the eye would be needed to rule out intraocular haemorrhages [41].

- Lateral medullary syndrome will require a thorough systemic evaluation to rule out diabetes mellitus, hypertension and heart disease. Complete blood work-up, cardiac investigations like electrocardiogram (ECG), echocardiography and carotid Doppler. CTA and MRA will provide a precise location of the infarct [42].

- In CCF, the prominence of the superior ophthalmic vein (SOV) and the diffuse enlargement of the extraocular muscles are demonstrated by CT and MRI. Additionally, orbital Doppler imaging can be used to assess abnormal flow patterns, especially in the SOV. To classify CCF and plan the mode of management, selective catheter DSA, CTA and MRA can be useful [43–45].

- The first step for investigating a stroke would be non-contrast CT to rule out haemorrhagic stroke. MRI with diffusion-weighted imaging (DWI) is required for evaluating posterior circulation strokes. It is mandatory to do a thorough clinical ophthalmic examination of visual acuity determination, pupillary exam, fundoscopy, and visual field testing [46, 47].

4. Visual rehabilitation

Vision rehabilitation is mandatory as vision loss can cause a major impact on the patient's life. Low vision therapy is important to treat and manage the symptoms of vision loss. Optical therapy incorporates the use of mirrors and prisms to enhance the patient's visual field. Strategies are devised to help the patients compensate and adapt to their visual impairment.

5. Recommendations

- Periodic radiographic imaging (either MRA, CT scan or conventional angiography) should be recommended at intervals to monitor the size and/or growth of the aneurysm in all cerebral artery aneurysm patients to avoid severe vision-threatening outcomes.

- There is general agreement to recommend cardiac monitoring, airway support and ventilatory assistance in the treatment of haemorrhagic and ischemic stroke patients.

- Strabismus surgery should be considered to correct the ocular misalignment associated with brainstem strokes, if not resolving on its own after 6 months.

- Visual rehabilitation can help make use of the remaining vision and other skills to increase independency.

- Role of an orthoptist is important to assess and treat the range of eye problems, pertaining to eye movements in cases of ophthalmoplegia.

6. Conclusions

Cerebral arterial circulation diseases are a complex group of diseases, which are confusing and hard to understand for neophyte residents. Understanding the cause and pathophysiology of these diseases (in a realistic way with the help of 3D animations), helps them to tackle these pathologies effectively [48]. In this chapter, we have used 3D animations and have taken the medical field from a field of theoretical curiosity into a world of animative reality.

Acknowledgements

We are grateful to Mr. Pragash Michael Raj - Department of Multimedia, Mahathma Eye Hospital Private Limited, Trichy, Tamil Nadu, India for his technical support throughout the making of this chapter and its illustrations. We sincerely thank Ms. Banasmita Mohanty for her support in proofreading the chapter.

Conflict of interest

The authors declare no conflict of interest.

Notes/thanks/other declarations

I (Dr. Prasanna Venkatesh Ramesh) owe a deep sense of gratitude to my daughters (Pranu and Hasanna) and family (in-laws) for all their prayers, support, and encouragement. Above all, I extend my heartfelt gratitude to all the patients who consented to the images which are utilised for this chapter.

I (Dr. Shruthy Vaishali Ramesh) want to thank my partner (Arul) for his constant support and encouragement during the process of creating this chapter.

I (Ms. Prajnya Ray) would like to offer my special thanks to Mr. Deepak Kumar Panda for his constant support and never-ending encouragement, and my parents for their support and motivation during the process of framing this chapter.

I (Mr. Aji Kunnath Devadas) want to thank my parents (Mr. Devadas K and Mrs. Sheeba Devadas) for their constant support and encouragement during the process of creating this chapter.

DOI: http://dx.doi.org/10.5772/intechopen.102846

Declaration of patient consent

In the form, the patient(s) has/have given his/her/their consent for his/her/their images and other clinical information to be reported in the chapter. The patients understand that their names and initials will not be published and due efforts will be made to conceal their identity, but anonymity cannot be guaranteed.

Nomenclature

3D	Three-dimensional
AVF	Arteriovenous Fistula
AVM	Arteriovenous Malformations
CCF	Carotid-Cavernous Fistula
CCM	Cerebral Cavernous Malformations
CN	Cranial Nerve
CT scan	Computed Tomography Scan
CTA	Computed Tomography Angiography
DSA	Digital Subtraction Angiography
DWI	Diffusion-Weighted Imaging
ECG	Electrocardiogram
ECHO	Echocardiography
INO	Internuclear Ophthalmoplegia
LGB	Lateral Geniculate Body
LMN	Lower Motor Neuron
LMS	Lateral Medullary Syndrome
LP	Lumbar Puncture
MLF	Medial Longitudinal Fasciculus
MRA	Magnetic Resonance Imaging Angiography
MRI	Magnetic Resonance Imaging
PCA	Posterior Cerebral Artery
PComA	Posterior Communicating Artery
PPRF	Paramedian Pontine Reticular Formation
SOV	Superior Ophthalmic Vein
TIA	Transient Ischemic Attack
TS	Terson's Syndrome
WEBINO	Wall-Eyed Bilateral Internuclear Ophthalmoplegia
WEMINO	Wall-Eyed Mono-Ocular Internuclear Ophthalmoplegia
XT	Exotropia

Author details

Prasanna Venkatesh Ramesh[1*], Shruthy Vaishali Ramesh[2], Prajnya Ray[3], Aji Kunnath Devadas[3], Tensingh Joshua[4], Anugraha Balamurugan[5], Meena Kumari Ramesh[2] and Ramesh Rajasekaran[6]

1 Department of Glaucoma and Research, Mahathma Eye Hospital Private Limited, Trichy, Tamil Nadu, India

2 Department of Cataract and Refractive Surgery, Mahathma Eye Hospital Private Limited, Trichy, Tamil Nadu, India

3 Department of Optometry and Visual Science, Mahathma Eye Hospital Private Limited, Trichy, Tamil Nadu, India

4 Mahathma Centre of Moving Images, Mahathma Eye Hospital Private Limited, Trichy, Tamil Nadu, India

5 Department of Vitreo-Retinal Surgery, Mahathma Eye Hospital Private Limited, Trichy, Tamil Nadu, India

6 Department of Paediatric Ophthalmology and Strabismus, Mahathma Eye Hospital Private Limited, Trichy, Tamil Nadu, India

*Address all correspondence to: email2prajann@gmail.com

References

[1] Cerebrovascular disease. Wikipedia [Internet]; 2021 [cited 2021 Dec 31]. Available from: https://en.wikipedia.org/w/index.php?title=Cerebrovascular_disease&oldid=1054526849

[2] Ramesh PV, Ray P, Ramesh SV, Devadas AK, Joshua T, Balamurugan A, et al. Cerebral arterial circulation: 3D augmented reality models and 3D printed puzzle models. In: Scerrati DA, Ricciardi DL, Dones DF, editors. Cerebral Circulation - Updates on Models, Diagnostics and Treatments of Related Diseases [Working Title] [Internet]. London: IntechOpen; 2022 [cited 2022 Feb 05]

[3] Ramesh PV, Aji K, Ray P, Ramesh SV, Balamurugan A, Ramesh MK, et al. Holistic integrative ophthalmology with multiplex imaging. TNOA Journal of Ophthalmic Science Research. 2021;**59**:420-424

[4] Ramesh SV, Ramesh PV. Photo quiz: Holistic integrative ophthalmology with multiplex imaging. TNOA Journal of Ophthalmic Science Research. 2020;**58**:334-335

[5] Ramesh SV, Ramesh PV. Photo Quiz Answers. TNOA Journal of Ophthalmic Science Research. 2020;**58**:336

[6] Ramesh SV, Ramesh PV, Ramesh MK, Padmanabhan V, Rajasekaran R. COVID-19-associated papilledema secondary to cerebral venous thrombosis in a young patient. Indian Journal of Ophthalmology. 2021;**69**:770-772

[7] Ramesh SV, Ramesh PV, Ray P, Balamurugan A, Madhanagopalan VG. Photo quiz: Holistic integrative ophthalmology with multiplex imaging - Part II. TNOA Journal of Ophthalmic Science Research. 2021;**59**:228-229

[8] Ramesh SV, Ramesh PV, Ray P, Balamurugan A, Madhanagopalan VG. Photo quiz answers. TNOA Journal of Ophthalmic Science Research. 2021;**59**:230

[9] Ramesh PV, Ray P, Aji K, Ramesh SV, et al. The COVID-19 Disease-Related And Vaccines Related Blood Clot Threat - What We Know So Far And Why Ophthalmologists Have To Be More Vigilant? Nix Journal of Clinical Case Reports. 100002

[10] Beck J, Rohde S, Berkefeld J, Seifert V, Raabe A. Size and location of ruptured and unruptured intracranial aneurysms measured by 3-dimensional rotational angiography. Surgical Neurology. 2006;**65**(1):18-25. discussion 25-27

[11] Dimopoulos VG, Fountas KN, Feltes CH, Robinson JS, Grigorian AA. Literature review regarding the methodology of assessing third nerve paresis associated with non-ruptured posterior communicating artery aneurysms. Neurosurgical Review. 2005;**28**(4):256-260

[12] Terson Syndrome: Don't Let It Go Unrecognized [Internet]. American Academy of Ophthalmology; 2018 [cited 2021 Oct 21]. Available from: https://www.aao.org/eyenet/article/terson-syndrome-dont-let-it-go-unrecognized

[13] Kim JS. Pure lateral medullary infarction: clinical-radiological correlation of 130 acute, consecutive patients. Brain. 2003;**126**(Pt 8):1864-1872

[14] Saleem FM, Das J. Lateral Medullary Syndrome. Treasure Island, FL: StatPearls Publishing; 2021 [cited 2021 Dec 4]. Available from: http://www.ncbi.nlm.nih.gov/books/NBK551670/

[15] Chaudhry IA, Elkhamry SM, Al-Rashed W, Bosley TM. Carotid cavernous fistula: Ophthalmological implications. Middle East African Journal of Ophthalmology. 2009;**16**(2):57-63

[16] Bowling B, Kanski JJ. Kanski's clinical ophthalmology: A systematic approach. 8th ed. Elsevier; 2016

[17] Modi P, Arsiwalla T. Cranial Nerve III Palsy [Internet]. Treasure Island (FL): StatPearls Publishing; 2021 [cited 2021 Nov 18]. Available from: http://www.ncbi.nlm.nih.gov/books/NBK526112/

[18] Khanam S, Sood G. Trochlear Nerve Palsy [Internet]. Treasure Island (FL): StatPearls Publishing; 2021 [cited 2021 Nov 11]. Available from: http://www.ncbi.nlm.nih.gov/books/NBK565850/

[19] Graham C, Mohseni M. Abducens Nerve Palsy [Internet]. Treasure Island (FL): StatPearls Publishing; 2021 [cited 2021 Nov 11]. Available from: http://www.ncbi.nlm.nih.gov/books/NBK482177/

[20] Khazaal O, Marquez DL, Naqvi IA. Foville Syndrome [Internet]. Treasure Island (FL): StatPearls Publishing; 2021 [cited 2021 Nov 12]. Available from: http://www.ncbi.nlm.nih.gov/books/NBK544268/

[21] Feroze KB, Patel BC. Parinaud Syndrome [Internet]. Treasure Island (FL): StatPearls Publishing; 2021 [cited 2021 Nov 12]. Available from: http://www.ncbi.nlm.nih.gov/books/NBK441892/

[22] Shields M, Sinkar S, Chan W, Crompton J. Parinaud syndrome: a 25-year (1991-2016) review of 40 consecutive adult cases. Acta Ophthalmologica. 2017;**95**(8):e792-e793

[23] Brodsky MC, Donahue SP, Vaphiades M, Brandt T. Skew deviation revisited. Survey of Ophthalmology. 2006;**51**(2):105-128

[24] Kim JS. Internuclear ophthalmoplegia as an isolated or predominant symptom of brainstem infarction. Neurology. 2004;**62**(9):1491-1496

[25] Feroze KB, Wang J. Internuclear Ophthalmoplegia [Internet]. Treasure Island (FL): StatPearls Publishing; 2021 [cited 2021 Nov 15]. Available from: http://www.ncbi.nlm.nih.gov/books/NBK441970/

[26] Shinoda K, Matsushita T, Furuta K, Isobe N, Yonekawa T, Ohyagi Y, et al. Wall-eyed bilateral internuclear ophthalmoplegia (WEBINO) syndrome in a patient with neuromyelitis optica spectrum disorder and anti-aquaporin-4 antibody. Multiple Sclerosis. 2011;**17**(7):885-887

[27] Jeon SB, Chung SJ, Ahn H, Lee J-H, Jung JM, Lee MC. Wall-Eyed Monocular Internuclear Ophthalmoplegia (WEMINO) with Contraversive Ocular Tilt Reaction. Journal of Clinical Neurology. 2005;**1**(1):101-103

[28] Xue F, Zhang L, Zhang L, Ying Z, Sha O, Ding Y. One-and-a-half syndrome with its spectrum disorders. Quantitative Imaging in Medicine and Surgery. 2017;**7**(6):691-697

[29] Mesina BVQ, Sosuan GMN, Reyes KB. Eight-and-a-half syndrome: a rare potentially life-threatening disease. GMS Ophthalmology Cases. 2018;**8**:Doc04

[30] Gómez Iglesias P, Sanesteban Beceiro E, Gómez Ruíz MN, Matías Guiu JA. Half and half syndrome as a presentation of multiple sclerosis. Neurología. 2021;**36**(3):246-248

[31] Topilow HW. Posterior internuclear ophthalmoplegia of Lutz. Annals of Ophthalmology. 1981;**13**(2):221-225

[32] Ashok A, Parthasarathi S, Ramesh PV. Diclofenac-induced papilledema. TNOA Journal of Ophthalmic Science and Research. 2021;**59**:199-201

[33] Shelton JB, Digre KB, Katz BJ, Warner JEA, Quigley EP. Chiasmal stroke in patient with atrial fibrillation and complete occlusion of right internal carotid artery. Journal of Neuro-Ophthalmology. 2012;**32**(2):189

[34] Fabian ID, Greenberg G, Huna-Baron R. Chiasmal stroke following open-heart surgery. Journal of Neuro-Ophthalmology. 2010;**30**(3):219-221

[35] Savino PJ, Paris M, Schatz NJ, Orr LS, Corbett JJ. Optic tract syndrome. A review of 21 patients. Archives of Ophthalmology. 1978;**96**(4):656-663

[36] De Vries TM, Aries MJH, De Groot JC, Bonte GJ, de Jong BM. A grid-like hemi-field defect following a lacunar infarct in the lateral geniculate nucleus. Clinical Neurology and Neurosurgery. 2012;**114**(3):278-280

[37] Pula JH, Yuen CA. Eyes and stroke: the visual aspects of cerebrovascular disease. Stroke and Vascular Neurology. 2017;**2**(4):210

[38] Glisson CC. Visual loss due to optic chiasm and retrochiasmal visual pathway lesions. Continuum (Minneap Minn). 2014;**20**(4 Neuro-Ophthalmology):907-921

[39] Cheng B, Forkert ND, Zavaglia M, Hilgetag CC, Golsari A, Siemonsen S, et al. Influence of stroke infarct location on functional outcome measured by the modified rankin scale. Stroke. 2014;**45**(6):1695-1702

[40] Gheewala G, Gadhia R, Surani SR, Ratnani I. Posterior Alien Hand Syndrome from Acute Ischemic Left Parietal Lobe Infarction. Cureus. 2019;**11**(10):e5828

[41] Terson Syndrome. 2020th ed. Thieme Verlag; 2020 [cited 2021 Oct 22]. Available from: https://www.thieme-connect.de/products/ebooks/lookinside/10.1055/b-0040-174266

[42] Nouh A, Remke J, Ruland S. Ischemic Posterior Circulation Stroke: A Review of Anatomy, Clinical Presentations, Diagnosis, and Current Management. Frontiers in Neurology. 2014;**5**:30

[43] Jindal G, Miller T, Raghavan P, Gandhi D. Imaging Evaluation and Treatment of Vascular Lesions at the Skull Base. Radiologic Clinics of North America. 2017;**55**(1):151-166

[44] Williams ZR. Carotid-Cavernous Fistulae: A Review of Clinical Presentation, Therapeutic Options, and Visual Prognosis. International Ophthalmology Clinics. 2018;**58**(2):271-294

[45] Meyers PM, Halbach VV, Dowd CF, Lempert TE, Malek AM, Phatouros CC, et al. Dural carotid cavernous fistula: definitive endovascular management and long-term follow-up. American Journal of Ophthalmology. 2002;**134**(1):85-92

[46] Merwick Á, Werring D. Posterior circulation ischemic stroke. BMJ. 2014;**348**:g3175

[47] Pollak L, Zehavi-Dorin T, Eyal A, Milo R, Huna-Baron R. Parinaud syndrome: Any clinicoradiological correlation? Acta Neurologica Scandinavica. 2017;**136**(6):721-726

[48] Ramesh PV, Aji K, Joshua T, Ramesh SV, Ray P, Raj PM, et al. Immersive photoreal new-age innovative gameful pedagogy for e-ophthalmology with 3D augmented reality. Indian Journal of Ophthalmology. 2022;**70**:275-280

Chapter 4

Measurement of Cerebral Circulation in Human

Sadegh Moradi, Hany Ferdinando, Aleksandra Zienkiewicz, Mariella Särestöniemi and Teemu Myllylä

Abstract

In this chapter, we review state-of-the-art non-invasive techniques to monitor and study cerebral circulation in humans. The measurement methods can be divided into two categories: direct and indirect methods. Direct methods are mostly based on using contrast agents delivered to blood circulation. Clinically used direct methods include single-photon emission computed tomography (SPECT), positron emission tomography (PET), magnetic resonance imaging (MRI) with contrast agents, xenon computed tomography (CT), and arterial spin labeling (ASL) MRI. Indirect techniques are based on measuring physiological parameters reflecting cerebral perfusion. The most commonly used indirect methods are near-infrared spectroscopy (NIRS), transcranial Doppler ultrasound (TCD), and phase-contrast MRI. In recent years, few more techniques have been intensively developed, such as diffuse correlation spectroscopy (DCS) and microwave-based techniques, which are still emerging as methods for cerebral circulation monitoring. In addition, methods combining different modalities are discussed and, as a summary, the presented techniques and their benefits for cerebral circulation will be compared.

Keywords: SPECT, PET, CT, ASL, MRI, NIRS, TCD, microwave, cerebral blood flow

1. Introduction

Human cerebral circulation involves a complex mechanisms [1] that attract researchers around the globe. The main purpose of cerebral circulation is to maintain energy and oxygen supply to the brain which is essential for normal brain function. The most important parameters reflecting cerebral circulation are cerebral blood flow (CBF), cerebral perfusion pressure (CPP), cerebrovascular resistance (CVR), and intracranial pressure (ICP). These have also an important role in diagnostics of many brain disorders, such as stroke, hemorrhage, head trauma, and carotid artery disease.

Human cerebral circulation monitoring can be performed using direct techniques, where CBF is directly measured, and indirect techniques that reflect relative changes in the cerebral circulation. At present, there are several imaging techniques that are commonly used in hospitals as stationary systems and require own imaging facilities due to complex imaging procedures. At first, these will be shortly introduced. Next, commonly known indirect methods are presented. These are typically portable devices and still are more commonly exploited in medical research. The chapter ends by presenting a few emerging methods that already show high potential for CBF monitoring but are still in the proof of concept phase.

2. Clinical stationary imaging devices

In this section, we present the most common cross-sectional imaging devices which can be utilized to measure CBF-related parameters. There are two nuclear medicine-based procedures, which are usually time-consuming, since radiotracers typically require several hours to accumulate in the tissue. These include positron emission tomography (PET) and computed tomography (CT). The first uses positron emitter radiotracers and the latter X-rays. During imaging, a narrow beam of positrons or X-ray irradiates the patient and quickly rotates around the head/body. Because of the harmful radiations, PET and CT techniques are usually used only for clinical diagnosis, although the radiation exposure is minimal. In general, these techniques do not provide continuous information on CBF [2]; however, they provide images with high spatial resolution and thus are used to detect possible cerebral circulation anatomy-related abnormalities.

Magnetic resonance imaging (MRI) is becoming the main technique for cross-sectional imaging of the brain since it is considered as a safe technique. In MRI, high-intensity alternative magnetic fields to align the protons in the imaged tissue. When the field is turned off, the protons are back to their initial direction by releasing stored energy. The amount of energy and the relaxation time is dependent on the chemical nature of the molecule and based on this information, the identity of the molecules can be determined [3]. The released energy is received by surrounding RF coils and prepared for data processing. Furthermore, functional MRI (fMRI) can detect magnetic changes associated with blood flow and thus can be exploited for imaging CBF, however, at lower spatial resolution than nuclear medicine-based techniques. In the following, the clinically available techniques are presented: PET, Single-Photon Emission CT (SPECT), Xenon CT (Xe-CT), and fMRI techniques based on contrast imaging that can be used for cerebral circulation imaging.

2.1 Positron emission tomography

PET can provide high-resolution images of cerebral circulation [4, 5]. It utilizes positron emitter radiotracers to generate high-quality images. The emitted positrons immediately collide with their antiparticles, electrons, then two gamma photons will be created. This process is called "annihilation". The gamma photos are irradiated in the same energies but in opposite directions with 180° different from each other, see **Figure 1**. The pair of photons are simultaneously captured by the surrounding detectors, and powerful signal processing can generate the reconstructed image based on the detected photons [7].

In order to provide a quantitative measure of CBF [8], the PET scanner needs special radio-markers for each measurement and uses ^{15}O-labeled water. The radiotracer is produced by a cyclotron and injected into the patient before scanning, which increases the complexity of PET measurement.

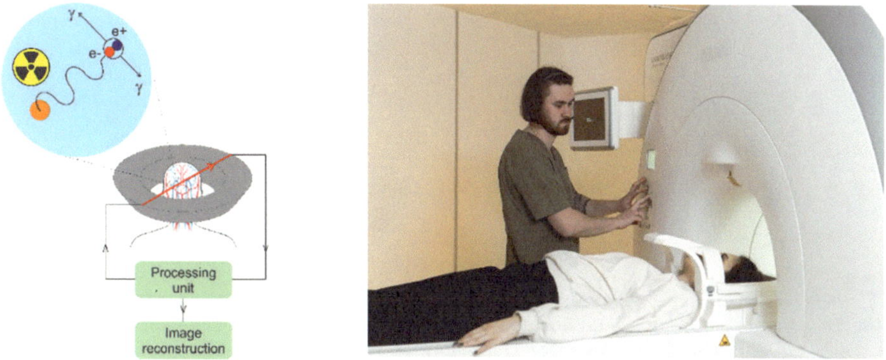

Figure 1.
The principle of PET scanning simplified from Ref. [6]. The emitted positron collides with an electron, then annihilation will happen. The basis of this phenomenon is the emission of two same-energy gamma photons in opposite directions. Finally, gamma detectors capture the photons and process them to reconstruct a 3D image. On the right, preparations to start brain imaging (Photo by MART PRODUCTION from pexels.com).

Clinical neurology usage of PET gradually started in the 1980s [9]. With ^{15}O tracers, it can provide essential information on patients with cerebral vascular disorders and information also on oxygen extraction fraction (OEF) and cerebral metabolic rate of oxygen $CRMO_2$. However, most techniques require an additional $C_{15}O$ scan for compensating cerebral blood volume (CBV) [10].

2.2 Single-photon emission computed tomography (SPECT)

Similar to PET, Single-Photon Emission Computed Tomography (SPECT), see **Figure 2**, is also a nuclear imaging technique utilizing a gamma-emitter radiotracer while PET employs positron emitters. In 1963, the first prototype of SPECT was presented by Edwards and Kuhl [12], but dedicated brain SPECT systems were introduced in 1980–1986, and then clinical brain imaging started immediately [13]. SPECT uses ^{99m}Tc radiotracer for CBF measurement [14]. The radiotracer penetrates through the blood-brain barrier (BBB) and diffuses in the brain tissue, proportionally to blood flow [15]. As a result, the gamma emission and SPECT scanner generate a comparative image. SPECT is a semi-quantitative CBF measurement technique and provides less spatial resolution compared to PET [16, 17].

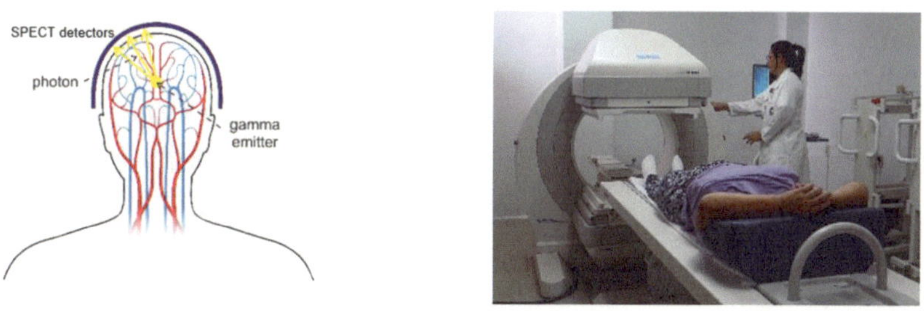

Figure 2.
SPECT device uses gamma-emitter radiotracers, which can be given by injection, inhalation, or orally. The SPECT detectors receive the gamma radiation and deliver the signal to the image processing and reconstruction unit [11]. The image on the right is courtesy of IAEA Imagebank.

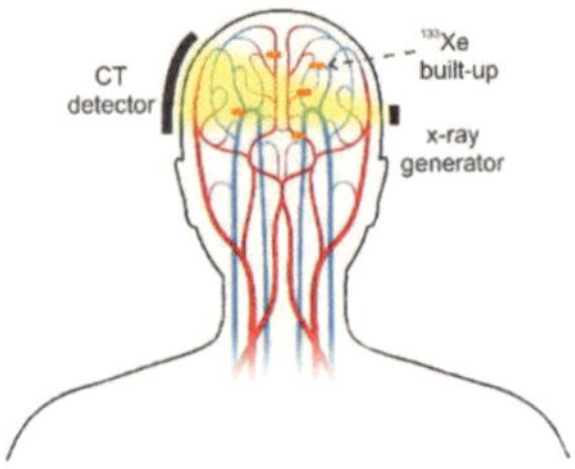

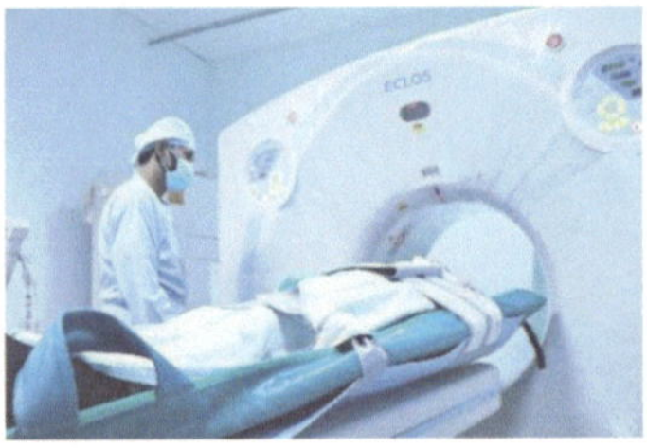

Figure 3.
Xe-CT system contains a rotating X-ray source and an array of detectors that generate a tomographic image. The inhaled xenon gas can partly block X-ray and provide quantitative indicators for CBF measurement. High-resolution Xe-CT CBF imaging (see on the right) takes about 10 min [14].

2.3 Xenon computed tomography (Xe-CT)

Xe-CT is one of the most accurate methods for obtaining quantitative CBF imaging. The system contains a rotating X-ray source and an array of detectors that generate a tomographic image of the brain or other organ [18], see **Figure 3**. The technology has been available since 1977, but its usage was not widespread until the 1990s. The scanning procedure is simple and quick and therefore is nowadays a commonly used clinical imaging device.

Xenon is an inert as well as radiopaque gas which can across the BBB and thus can reach deep brain tissue. Moreover, due to the short half-life of ^{131}Xe, it delivers a low amount of dose to the patient and allows multiple scans during CBF measurement [19]. However, a limitation of this technique is difficulty with the assessment of CBF in the posterior fossa and infratentorial region. The bones of the upper cervical spine, cranium, and facial structures produce artifacts on baseline CT images and make interpretation of blood flow difficult [20, 21]. Another limitation is the high sensitivity to motion artifacts. If a patient is not able to stay still during the scanning sequence, when xenon gas is being administered, it reduces the reliability of the blood flow information.

2.4 Arterial spin labeling MRI

Arterial spin labeling (ASL) is a non-invasive imaging technique using standard MRI. The measurement of blood flow is based on magnetically labeled arterial blood water protons that are used as tracers [22]. The techniques are suitable also for imaging children as the use of radioactive and contrast agents can be restricted. The ASL method was originally proposed by Williams and his colleagues when they attempted to measure CBF from rats using water as a diffusible tracer [23]. In 1994, the method was extended to human brain imaging [24].

The main idea was to provide the same image with and without magnetization of the blood flow [25], by giving radiofrequency pulses to invert or saturate the water protons in blood [23]. With the fact that the relaxation time of water in the blood is about 1–2 s, the brain will not be overflowed with spin-labeled water [24, 26]. By subtracting the image with magnetization from the other one, it results in CBF information.

Different techniques of ASL including continuous arterial spin labeling (CASL) [23], pseudo-continuous ASL (PCASL), and velocity-selective ASL (VS-ASL) are possible. The two latest methods were developed to solve problems and challenges encountered in CASL. Modified ASL techniques, such as territorial ASL (TASL) can be used for imaging

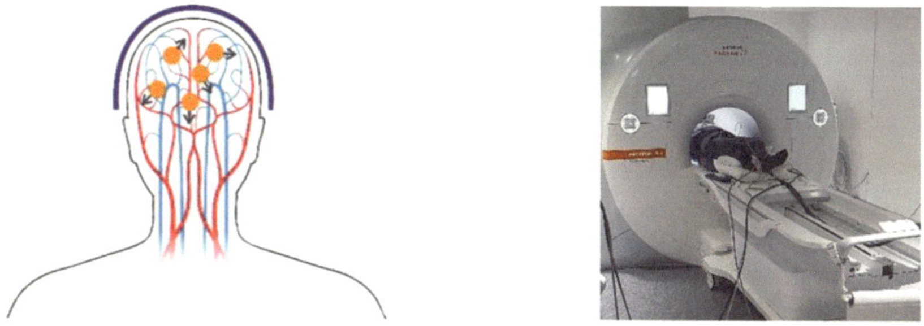

Figure 4.
In MRI, the magnet firstly applies a powerful field to align the protons. When it is turned off, the protons release their energies and turn back to their initial state. At this stage, head coils receive the released energy. On the right, performing fMRI brain imaging in Oulu University Hospital.

collateral and visualization of perfusion of individual arteries [27–29], whereas ASL at multiple delay times (Tis) is capable of depicting areas with low CBF (**Figure 4**) [30].

ASL-MRI holds high potential. For instance, patients with ischemic stroke suffer from decreased cerebral perfusion [31]. ASL has been used to assess various perfusions, e.g., hemispheric perfusion deficits, post-ischemic hyperperfusion, or perfusion-diffusion mismatches [32]. Furthermore, several studies in dementia employed ASL to assess regional hyperperfusion from patients with Alzheimer's disease (AD), front temporal dementia, and mild cognitive impairment [26, 33]. The results were in line with the previous studies using PET and SPECT. Sandson et al. used ASL to study parieto-occipital and temporo-occipital among controls and AD subjects [34]. They could separate these groups based on the decreased perfusion in those regions. ASL technique was also found useful in epilepsy studies as the abnormal tissue had a lower metabolic rate and blood flow than the other [35]. It was suspected that the hypoperfusion interictal pattern was associated with neuronal loss, although the mechanism behind the hypoperfusion interictal is still unknown. Based on a study during the interictal state, hypoperfusion occurred in the involved cortex [36].

2.5 Contrast-enhanced MRI (CE-MRI)

As ASL MRI uses magnetically labeled arterial blood water protons as tracers [22], contrast-enhanced MRI (CE-MRI) employs pharmaceutical tracers to enhance image quality. This improves the visibility of the internal structures and emphasizes the difference between normality and abnormalities in brain tissue e.g., tumors or disrupted blood-brain barrier, and can enhance diagnosis and staging of malignancies, treatment planning, and monitoring the response to therapy [37]. Other current applications of CE-MRI include the assessment of vascular disease (stroke and vascular malformations) and monitoring of inflammatory, neurodegenerative and infectious diseases. Perfusion imaging using CE-MRI is used in brain tumor imaging, based on the principle of increased tumor vascularity. CE-MRI technique has been developed with variations such as dynamic contrast-enhanced (DCE) MRI and dynamic susceptibility contrast (DSC) MRI, which also have a role in tumor imaging to assess vascular permeability and angiogenesis, respectively [37].

Young et al. pioneered the use of ferric chloride as the contrast agent in the MRI for gastrointestinal track in 1981 [38]. Since 1988, the most commonly used in clinical practice are contrast agents with the lanthanide ion gadolinium (III) (Gd^{3+}), which were introduced to evaluate BBB disruption and vascular features with MR imaging.

Gd^{3+} possesses a high magnetic moment and is the most stable ion with unpaired electrons [39]. Several different variations of Gd^{3+} chelates are used for MRI contrast, often described under the group name of Gd-based contrast agents (GBCAs).

When using GBCAs the T1 or T2 relaxation times of nearby water protons are shortened; as a result, T1-weighted images have an increased signal intensity, while T2-weighted images signal intensity is reduced [39]. Contrast agents from the second group may contain e.g., transition metal manganese (Mn^{2+}), which has been suggested as being particularly effective for functional brain imaging, as it enters cells through calcium channels [40]. In general, these agents are injected systemically and enhance the overall image quality, without focusing on a specific area.

Despite the excellent quality obtained by using GBCAs in MRI imaging, the method still requires development, and its main challenge is the toxicity of the used substances. Gadolinium-based contrast agents were initially considered entirely safe, but eventually in 2006 were associated with nephrogenic systemic fibrosis and significant negative consequences in certain vulnerable patients, particularly for patients with impaired renal functionality [41]. Persons with normal kidney function have not been thought to be at risk, although some amounts of gadolinium can remain in the organs. Accumulation of gadolinium in the body is still being investigated. The long-term effects of retained gadolinium are unknown. For this reason, there are ongoing investigations into alternative compounds which could be used as contrast agents. Several types of gadolinium-free contrast agents have been investigated, for instance, organic radical contrast agents (ORCAs), which have low cytotoxicity and high biodegradability, reducing the potential for side effects [42]. However, further investigation and performance development need to be performed before newer contrast agents can be used in clinical practice.

3. Portable devices (indirect methods)

3.1 Functional near-infrared spectroscopy

Functional near-infrared spectroscopy (fNIRS) refers to an optics-based measurement method using two or more wavelengths in the near-infrared (NIR) range (650–950 nm), see **Figure 5**. When NIR light illuminates sculp, it experiences scattering and absorption. A part of the incident light reaches the brain cortex and reflects and scatters back to sculp which can be detected by a sensitive photodetector. When

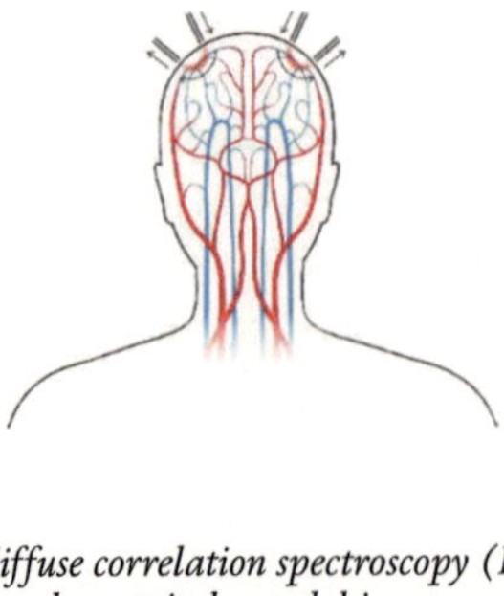

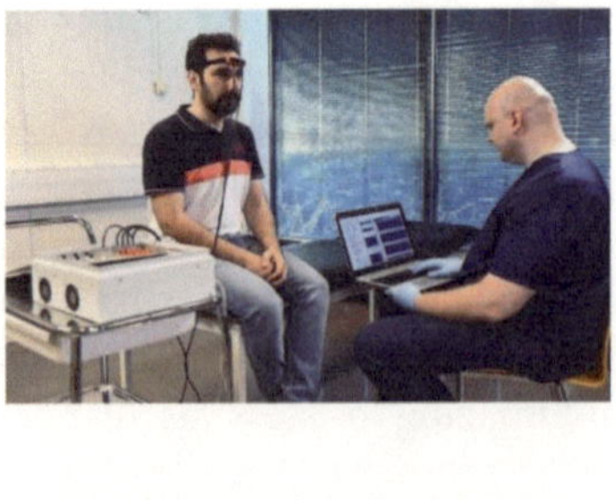

Figure 5.
fNIRS and diffuse correlation spectroscopy (DCS) are two optical technologies for human brain monitoring that are sensitive to changes in hemoglobin concentrations and blood flow, respectively. Typically, light source and detector are placed at a distance of 3–4 cm from each other in order to form an optical measurement volume that reaches 1–2 cm depth. As illustrated on the left, the measurement volume can be shown as a banana-shaped area. On the right, performing fNIRS measurement in Oulu University Hospital.

using at least one wavelength on both sides of the isosbestic point at ~810 nm, cerebral hemodynamics can be quantified based on the modified Beer-Lambert law [43]. The most common signals to read are oxy- and deoxy-hemoglobin, abbreviated here as HbO and HbR, respectively, while MRI can only provide blood-oxygenation-level-dependent (BOLD), which is basically HbR [44]. Furthermore, fNIRS can be used to measure cerebral blood volume (CBV) based on quantifying HbT [45], various additional hemodynamic parameters [46–49], and cytochrome c oxide [50].

fNIRS provides a more affordable solution when compared to devices presented in the clinical stationary imaging devices sub-section. Several measurement principles in fNIRS include continuous wave (cwNIRS), time-domain (TD-NIRS), frequency-domain (FD-NIRS), and frequency-coded NIRS systems [51]. The technique is fully safe and can also be realized as a wearable continuous monitoring setup. For example, SPECT and PET cannot measure dynamic changes in cerebral circulation whereas fNIRS is capable of that [52], however, it suffers from low spatial resolution. Kusaka et al. [46] emphasized that monitoring of cerebral circulation in infants is needed in general clinical practice, however, for this purpose e.g., MRI or PET are not suitable. They evaluated fNIRS to measure oxygen saturation (ScO_2), CBV, CBF, and cerebral metabolic rate of oxygen to study cerebral circulation in infants and concluded that fNIRS is a potential technique for bedside brain monitoring in a neo-natal intensive care unit (NICU).

3.2 Diffuse correlation spectroscopy

DCS is a non-invasive method based on speckle fluctuations caused by the interference of the multiple and random paths of photons traveling in tissue. The speckle fluctuations are mostly caused by the motion of red blood cells and recorded signal fluctuations thus reflecting blood flow in the microvasculature. For this, a blood flow index (BFI) value is provided. The measurement setup is similar to fNIRS, see **Figure 5**, but DCS requires the use of laser light with a long coherence length for detection of temporal speckle effects. It measures the decorrelation time scale of the intensity fluctuations of the scattered light, which relates to the motion of moving scattering centers, mostly consisting of red blood cells in CBF [53]. The principle of the DCS technique is well described in several papers [54–56]. This still a relatively new method shows increasingly high potential for human cerebral circulation monitoring, especially for clinical monitoring newborns [57–59]. At present, portable, low-cost DCS setups are being developed and apparently will be in near future utilized in clinics and patient bedsides [55, 60]. These will be most likely used combined with fNIRS to provide comprehensive information on cerebral hemodynamics and circulation [61].

3.3 Transcranial Doppler ultrasound

Transcranial Doppler (TCD) is a non-invasive method used for the measurement of blood flow velocity within the large arteries of the circle of Willis. It was introduced in 1982 by R. Aaslid, who tested the applicability of existing range-gated ultrasound Doppler instruments in cerebral circulation monitoring [62]. It was initially suggested as a method for the detection of vasospasm following subarachnoid hemorrhage and for evaluating cerebral circulation in occlusive disease of the carotid and vertebral arteries. However, thanks to constant experiments and advances of the technique, current applications are extensive and TCD is widely used in neurological disorders diagnosis and monitoring. Moreover, the development of transcranial color-coded duplex (TCCD) examination provided a possibility of direct visualization of the cerebral anatomy vessels and enabled accuracy improvement as well as broadening the scope of applications.

Ultrasound-based techniques measure the frequency change in pulse reflecting from the particular structure. When used in medical applications, it allows defining the speed of the red blood cells in vessels and arteries, as well as the flow direction. The ultrasound probe is emitting the pulse of known frequency toward the flowing blood, then the same probe is detecting the pulse-echo. The frequency of the ultrasound pulses used in TCD is relatively low (2.0–2.5 MHz), as it needs to penetrate through the skull. To reduce signal attenuation, the probe is placed above thinner parts of the skull (insonation windows), such as the transtemporal, transforaminal, transorbital, and transcervical windows. Each of the windows allows better access to different branches of the circle of Willis: *transtemporal window*: terminal internal carotid artery (ICA), middle cerebral artery (MCA), anterior cerebral artery (ACA), posterior cerebral artery (PCA), and communicating arteries, *transorbital window*: ophthalmic artery (OA) and ICA siphon (carotid siphon), *suboccipital window*: vertebral artery (VA) and basilar artery (BA); *submandibular window*: extracranial ICA and common carotid artery.

Figure 6 shows how the TCD probe is placed over a transtemporal window, with an ultrasound penetrating toward the brain vasculature.

TCD does not measure the diameter (or cross-sectional area) of the artery, due to low penetration of the ultrasound. Thus, the actual value provided in this technique is the relative velocity in the artery of interest, calculated using the formula for the Doppler shift [14]. With the assumption that vessel diameter (and insonation angle) remains constant, detected changes in blood flow equal to changes in CBF. Consequently, vessel diameter stability affects estimates of CBF using TCD, which should be especially considered during interventions. In order to approximate flow velocity as an estimate of flow and minimize the method inaccuracy, different indices are calculated, such as the pulsatility index (PI) and the resistance index (RI).

Conventional TCD enables the measurement of blood flow velocity and its changes with high temporal resolution (above 10 Hz). However, correct probe placement and the identification of the vessel require a skilled person, as only blood flow velocity changes in time are visible. This TCD type is non-duplex: there is no imaging available, and the artery identification is done based on audible Doppler shift and the spectral display. Applications of TCD include diagnosis of acute ischemic stroke, vasospasm, traumatic brain injury, measurement of cerebrovascular reserve capacity, examination of autoregulation and neurovascular coupling, microembolus

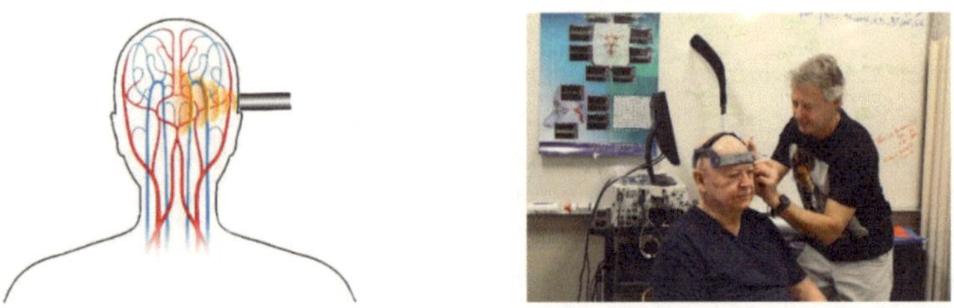

Figure 6.
TCD probe placement (on the left) over the transtemporal window is the easiest to access and the most widely used in clinical practice. The image on the right, showing TCD measurement, is courtesy of Journalism School Newswire.

detection, ultrasound enhanced thrombolysis, assessment of increased intracranial pressure (ICP), detection of the stop of brain circulation in brain death, and monitoring of cerebral circulation during carotid or heart surgery [63]. The accuracy of the conventional TCD can be improved by using an ultrasound contrast agent in contrast-enhanced TCD (c-TCD) [64]. This technique may also improve the detection of flows in non-conclusive TCD, however, its limitations are availability and cost [64].

Adding imaging features to the TCD technique improved the measurement's quality and broadened the scope of applications. Transcranial color-coded duplex (TCCD) uses a combination of pulsed-wave Doppler ultrasound and a cross-sectional view of the area of insonation. It provides real-time visualization of measured intracranial arteries in relation to various anatomic locations, thus simplifying corrections of insonation angles and improving measurement accuracy. The color-coded Doppler also presents the direction of the flow in relation to the probe. TCCD is mostly used in hemodynamic assessment, but is applicable in many other neurocritical care scenarios, such as detection of intra- and extra-axial intracranial hematomas, midline shift, hydrocephaly, cerebral tumors, cerebral aneurysms, as well as investigation of arteriovenous malformations and cerebral parenchyma [63, 64].

There are several unquestionable advantages to the TCD technique, namely its non-invasive nature, the fact that it is radiation-free, and high temporal resolution. The technique is portable, relatively low-cost, and widely available. However, it is important to note several major limitations. TCD measurement has poor spatial resolution and thus is limited to large basal arteries. It can only provide an index of global rather than local CBF velocity [65]. Also, recorded values are relative. The measurement can only be performed through the insonation windows, and it is essential to choose the appropriate one. In some cases, the chosen insonation window might be inaccessible (up to 15% of the population), e.g., due to thick bone structure causing the signal amplitude reduction. It has been observed especially among older or female patients. Another limitation is the influence of the insonation angle, as the wrong angle can affect in recording inaccurate velocities. Therefore, careful probe placement is crucial and might be challenging, especially in conventional TCD, where operator dependency is a significant drawback itself.

4. Emerging methods

There are several new methods in development that potentially can be exploited in CBF studies. In addition, combining different techniques can provide better, more comprehensive information on cerebral circulation.

4.1 Ultrasound-tagged NIRS

Ultrasound-Tagged (UT) NIRS is a relatively new technique based on the acousto-optic effect where photons are modulated or tagged at the acoustic frequency [66]. Basically, a low-power ultrasound transducer is used to modulate the high coherent near infra-red photons, then due to blood flow, the Doppler effect will rise [67]. In other words, when the tagged photons collide with blood content, a frequency shift will be observed, as an indicator of blood flow. The UT-NIRS system employs both optical contrasts as well as ultrasound resolution to provide a deep CBF measurement, while other optical CBF techniques can measure blood flow in the outer part of the cerebrum [2]. Moreover, UT-NIRS is a real-time technique. Measurement depth can be adjusted by changing the focus point of the US transducer introduced by Tsalach et al. [2]. UT-NIRS can provide a cerebral flow index (CFI), a unitless and non-calibrated number from 0 to 100, reflecting CBF. Compared to fNIRS, the UT-NIRS technique has the capability of detection of intracerebral blood flow variation [68]. However, further studies and validation of its measurement accuracy still need to be conducted [66].

4.2 Microwave-based methods

The usability of microwave-based techniques has been studied for different medical diagnosis and monitoring applications for years since they could enable safe, reliable, low-power and low-cost, portable solutions which could be used also outside the hospitals. Besides, microwaves enable screening of the whole head, especially at lower microwave frequencies. Microwave-based techniques have been actively studied e.g., for detection of brain hemorrhages and strokes [69–73], brain water dynamics [74], tumors [75, 76]. Recently, microwave techniques have also been recognized to have the potential for monitoring cerebral circulation [77–81].

There are two approaches for microwaves-based cerebral circulation monitoring: In the first approach, the microwave-based technique is used to measure temperature and conductivity changes in the tissues which are caused by the changes in blood flow, see **Figure 7a**. Another approach is based on detecting changes in the blood volume which directly corresponds to the blood flow, see **Figure 7b**. The basic idea of these techniques is briefly described in the following subsections.

4.2.1 Detection of changes in temperature and conductivity

Microwave radiometry can be used to sense thermal radiation (electromagnetic noise) emitted in the microwave frequency spectrum by any material above absolute zero temperature. The thermal radiation is received by one or several sensitive antennas and converted, with proper calibration, into a measure of absolute temperature taken from a weighted average of the antenna's radiation pattern [82–85]. The basic idea of passive temperature sensing with microwaves is illustrated in **Figure 7a**. There are several studies on the non-invasive temperature measurement of the human brain which were originally targeted for observing the brain recovering from hypothermia [86, 87].

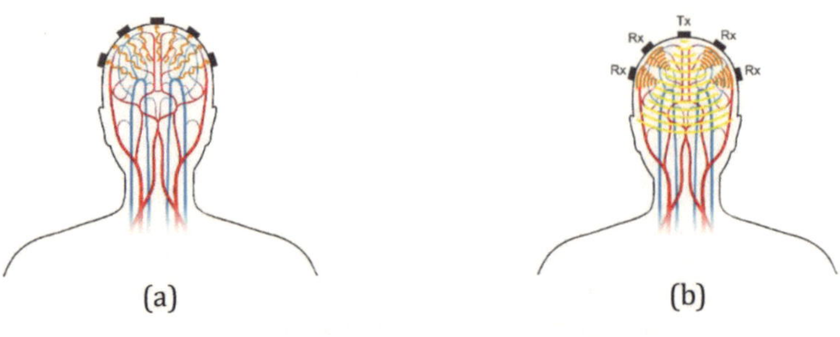

Figure 7.
(a) Passive microwave radiometry multi-antenna setup for monitoring cerebral circulation through temperature changes. The sensitive antennas are placed around the head for sensing the radiation. The received signals from the antenna ports are fed to a radiometer, which expresses changes in voltage. (b) Transmitter-receiver multiantenna setup for detecting changes in blood volume using reflected wave analysis: Tx antenna transmits microwaves and several Rx antennas are placed around head detecting signals reflected from tissue boundaries. ToF analysis indicates distances from different tissue borders detecting hence also blood volume changes.

Furthermore, fluid movements within an organ produce an elevation in the thermal conductivity, which is approximately a linear function of flow within the organ [88].

Recently, it has been recognized that measuring local changes in temperature and conductivity can be applied to estimate changes in blood flow or volume [77]. Various experiments, conducted both with tissue-mimicking phantoms as well as with human volunteers, have verified the contribution of microwave radiometry to temperature distribution imaging as well as tracking the changes in conductivity.

The most recent study in this field presents a new prototype of a passive microwave radiometry monitoring device for detecting changes in the temperature and the conductivity using four unipolar elliptical on-body antennas [77]. The sensitive antennas are placed around the head for sensing the radiation. The received signals from the four antenna ports are fed to a custom-made radiometer operating at 1.5 GHz, which is a suitable frequency to provide sufficient penetration of microwave radiation into the head tissue. Besides, the use of multiple antennas around the biological body enhances the in-depth detection ability as well as the sensitivity of the system. The experimental results presented in [77] prove that the system can sense local temperature or conductivity changes at a distance up to 5 cm in a brain phantom. The increased blood flow was indicated as 0.2–0.4 mV changes in the radiometer. More comprehensive studies on the accuracy of this method on exact blood flow measurements have not yet been published.

4.2.2 Detection of changes in blood volume

An increase in cerebral circulation can be observed as increased blood volume in the active brain areas, which can also be monitored in microwaves by detecting changes in blood volume with the analysis of electromagnetic (EM) propagation between the antennas located around the head. The technique is based on the physical phenomenon of EM propagation on the boundary between two media with different impedances: as the EM wave, transmitted from the transmitter antenna (Tx) encounters the border between two tissues, the fraction of the energy will be reflected and the remaining fraction will be propagated further deeper inside the tissue, as presented in **Figure 7b**. The time of flight (ToF) of the reflected wave can be measured with several sensitive receiver antennas (Rx), indicating the distance from the object that caused the reflection. Hence, if the local changes in blood volume inside the brain can be detected precisely enough with the analysis of the signals reflected from different head tissues, it can be indicated which parts of the brain are active at a time.

Originally, detection of the changes in blood volume in the brain area was applied for the detection of brain hemorrhage [72, 73]. The idea was further extended in [81] for initial blood circulation detection studies using a single chip implementation of an ultra-wideband impulse radar. Although the presented experimental setup did not reach in the required level of accuracy, it showed that UWB impulse radar is a promising technique for brain imaging and monitoring applications and inspired several new studies on higher-resolution brain activity monitoring [78–80, 89].

The recently presented idea to increase resolution in cerebral circulation monitoring is to provide diversity either using (a) antenna pattern reconfiguration or (b) Tx-signal waveform variation. Ojaroudi et al. [78] presented a study on applying these two diversity techniques for functional microwave imaging using an antenna array radar setup. Both diversity techniques have advantages in increasing either resolution, contrast, or target localization. In general, frequency selection and the properties of the antennas play a significant role in terms of achieved resolution and propagation depth [78, 81, 89]. Furthermore, the use of novel localization algorithms presented e.g., in [79] can further improve the resolution in brain imaging and hence also in detection of blood circulation. The above-mentioned techniques are recently published in initial studies on applying microwaves for cerebral circulation monitoring. More comprehensive studies on the accuracy of these methods on exact blood flow measurements have not yet been published.

5. Combining different methods

Simultaneous measurement using different techniques is increasingly being utilized in both research and clinical practice [90], since it allows a broader view on human physiology and underlying mechanisms. Brain studies can particularly benefit from a multimodal approach, because of the connection between neuronal activity and cerebral blood flow. Combining hemodynamic measurements with neuroimaging enables analysis of their dynamics in relation to each other and brain function, as well as it can provide complementary information on the relationship between systemic blood flow and influence on cerebral hemodynamics. On the other hand, combining modalities with different working principles enables to benefit from strong features present in each of them; an example can be combining the modality with high temporal resolution and modality with high spatial resolution. It might also be used as an alternative to methods of high cost, or to validate the accuracy of other measurement methods [47]. Not all of the modalities can be combined though, due to problems with compatibility. For instance, systems with ferromagnetic materials cannot be used within MRI environments [47] because of a large static magnetic field [91] whereas magnetoencephalography (MEG) is easily disturbed by electromagnetic interferences [92]. Thus, it is crucial to analyze the safety of the combined use of the devices before the measurements are conducted. In the following several combination techniques are listed, illustrating how multimodal measurements can be employed, depending on the signal/feature of interest.

Combining fNIRS with fMRI allows to study cerebral blood oxygenation during brain activation. fNIRS provides the benefit of accurate temporal resolution, whereas MRI performs with great spatial accuracy. Accurate anatomical information obtained using MRI enables to estimate NIR light propagation in the human head through different tissue layers [90]. On the other hand, fNIRS can measure complementary parameters (such as HbR and HbO), enabling estimation of the cerebral metabolic rate of oxygen.

Rostrup et al. [93] compared ΔHbO and ΔHbR from fNIRS with DCBV and DCBF changes from PET during various respiratory conditions. The values of DCBV from NIRS were similar to those from PET, but with much smaller magnitudes. Thus, fNIRS has the potential for cerebral circulation studies. Eke et al. [45] assess CBV based on the HbT concentration using a commercial multiwavelength fNIRS measured from the forehead. The periodogram of HbT was obtained from 0.000122 to 1 Hz using fast Fourier transform. Based on the fractal analysis on this periodogram to assess the self-similarity, its pattern started to change at a certain frequency, called as cut-off frequency. Interestingly, the range from minimum to the cut-off frequencies is narrower and narrower as age increases. Within female subjects, the pre- and post-menopausal age groups show different behavior. However, there is no significant difference between male and female subjects. They found a strong correlation between CBV changes measured by PET and HbT changes from NIRS.

TCD can be targeted to detect the increase in blood flow velocity in a specific vessel. However, due to poor spatial resolution, it is impossible to distinguish, if these changes are caused by the local or global increase in CBF. Using TCD simultaneously with fNIRS could improve overall spatial accuracy, due to the information on regional cerebral oxygenation provided by fNIRS [94, 95].

Furthermore, combining standard blood pulse measurement methods with brain activity monitoring can be used to investigate the interconnections between CBF and systemic circulation. It is a setup used e.g., in studies on cerebral autoregulation/ cerebral reactivity. Systemic blood flow can be tracked using invasive or non-invasive monitors. If the study is performed in the MRI chamber, it is necessary to use MRI-compatible blood pulsation tracking, e.g., utilizing fiber optics-based equipment [96].

Respiration measurement using e.g., pulse oximetry is often combined with brain monitoring methods such as fNIRS during sleep studies [97, 98]. Studies on cerebral hemodynamics during sleep are performed e.g., in order to assess the influence of various sleep-disordered breathing events (such as apnea) on the brain, as well as to understand the physiological and pathological mechanisms responsible for respiratory events during sleep.

The above-mentioned combined methods present just examples of using different measurement techniques simultaneously to emphasize its potential. However, more does not necessarily always mean better. Multiple metrics resulting from measuring with several techniques can be difficult to interpret, especially in clinical settings [99]. A method of data interpretation and analysis should also be planned when performing multimodal measurements. Understanding the benefits and drawbacks of available techniques will help to design the combination best suited for the pursued goals.

6. Summary

Table 1 compares the presented techniques used for monitoring cerebral circulation, particularly their output, resolution, and cost.

Clinical stationary imaging devices have the high spatial resolution, but the temporal resolution is usually relatively low. fMRI, for example, has low temporal resolution due to hemodynamic response time, which is much slower than the underlying neural process [100]. This problem has been solved by manipulating event-related stimuli and applying appropriate analysis methods [101].

Portable devices generally offer relatively low cost and rely on the indirect methods, which must be validated carefully. They are commonly suitable for bedside and continuous measurements, even for daily use. Particularly, optic-based methods have already shown their high potential for cerebral circulation studies. The penetration depth and spatial accuracy, however, are limited. TCD technique is non-invasive, radiation-free, and provides high temporal resolution. The device is widely available and of relatively low cost. However, the measurement has poor spatial resolution and provides only relative values on blood flow velocity. Monitoring with non-duplex TCD is also highly dependent on the skills of the operator. Insonation windows might be inaccessible for some patients, in which case the measurement cannot be performed.

There are several emerging techniques that can offer promising techniques for developing portable, low-cost, and safe devices for cerebral circulation monitoring. In particular, published initial feasibility studies show that functional microwave-based approaches show high potential. The benefit of cerebral circulation monitoring by detecting changes in the brain temperature/conductivity is the simplicity: the passive

Technology	Principle	Output	Temporal resolution	Spatial resolution	Cost
SPECT	Nuclear imaging technique utilizing a gamma-emitter radiotracer	3D image	Low	High	High
PET	Positron emitter radioactive tracers	3D image	Very low	High	High
ASL-MRI	Magnetically labeled water proton as tracers	3D image	Low	High	High
CT	Rotating x-ray beam	3D image	Low	High	High
fNIRS	Optic-based method	HbO, HbR, water, lipid	High	Low	Low
DCS	Optic-based method	Blood flow index	High	Low	Low
TCD	Ultrasound	Blood flow	High	Low	Low
Microwave	1. Sensing temperature and conductivity changes with mw antennas 2. Measuring signals reflected from the tissue boundaries	1. Temperature and conductivity changes, also converted to a voltage 2. Blood volume and images	High	Still unspecified	Medium or low

Table 1.
Comparison of selected techniques.

system just monitors the natural radiation and converts it to temperature values or voltage. The deficiency of this technique is the lack of accuracy in terms of the monitored area. However, the use of several antennas can improve accuracy clearly. The advantage of cerebral circulation monitoring by detecting changes in the blood volume is the possibility for higher resolution and localization accuracy, especially if advanced antennas, diversity techniques, and developed algorithms are utilized. The deficiency is the increased computational complexity in signal processing, which may require more expensive computers or distributed computing.

Acknowledgements

This work was supported by the Academy of Finland (grant 318347) and Academy of Finland Profi6 funding, 6G-Future Sustainable Society (University of Oulu), and Infotech Oulu.

Author details

Sadegh Moradi[1*], Hany Ferdinando[2], Aleksandra Zienkiewicz[1], Mariella Särestöniemi[2,3] and Teemu Myllylä[1,2]

1 Optoelectronics and Measurement Techniques Research Unit, University of Oulu, Oulu, Finland

2 Research unit of Medical Imaging, Physics and Technology, University of Oulu, Oulu, Finland

3 Center for Wireless Communications, University of Oulu, Oulu, Finland

*Address all correspondence to: sadegh.moradi@oulu.fi

References

[1] Panerai RB. Complexity of the human cerebral circulation. Philosophical Transactions of the Royal Society A: Mathematical, Physical and Engineering Sciences. 2009;**367**(1892):1319-1336

[2] Tsalach A, Schiffer Z, Ratner E, Breskin I, Zeitak R, Shechter R, et al. Depth selective acousto-optic flow measurement. Biomedical Optics Express. 2015. Available from: https://www.osapublishing.org/viewmedia.cfm?uri=boe-6-12-4871&seq=0&html=true;**6**(12):4871-4886 [cited 2021 Dec 14]

[3] Scherzinger AL, Hendee WR. Basic principles of magnetic resonance imaging—an update. Western Journal of Medicine. 1985;**143**(6):782-792

[4] Rostami E, Engquist H, Enblad P. Imaging of cerebral blood flow in patients with severe traumatic brain injury in the neurointensive care. Frontiers in Neurology. 2014;**5**:114

[5] Lin W, Celik A, Derdeyn C, An H, Lee Y, Videen T, et al. Quantitative measurements of cerebral blood flow in patients with unilateral carotid artery occlusion: A PET and MR study. Journal of Magnetic Resonance Imaging. 2001;**14**(6):659-667

[6] Langner J. Development of a Parallel Computing Optimized Head Movement Correction Method in Positron Emission Tomography (Thesis). Dresden, Germany: Technische Universität Dresden; 2003

[7] Townsend D. Physical principles and technology of clinical PET imaging. Annals of the Academy of Medicine, Singapore. 2004;**33**(2):133-145

[8] Derdeyn CP. Positron emission tomography imaging of cerebral ischemia. Neuroimaging Clinics of North America. 2005;**15**(2):341-350

[9] Coleman RE, Delbeke D, Guiberteau MJ, Conti PS, Royal HD, Weinreb JC, et al. Concurrent PET/CT with an integrated imaging system: Intersociety dialogue from the joint working group of the American College of Radiology, the Society of Nuclear Medicine, and the Society of Computed Body Tomography and Magnetic Resonance. Journal of the American College of Radiology. 2005;**2**(7):568-584

[10] Kudomi N, Hirano Y, Koshino K, Hayashi T, Watabe H, Fukushima K, et al. Rapid quantitative CBF and $CMRO_2$ measurements from a single PET scan with sequential administration of dual-15 O-labeled tracers. Journal of Cerebral Blood Flow & Metabolism. 2013;**33**(3):440-448

[11] Tsui BMW, Zhao X, Frey EC, McCartney WH. Quantitative single-photon emission computed tomography: Basic and clinical considerations. Seminars in Nuclear Medicine. 1994;**24**(1):38-65

[12] Kuhl DE, Edwards RQ. Image separation radioisotope scanning. Radiology. 1963;**80**:653-661

[13] Rogers WL, Clinthorne NH, Stamos J, Koral KF, Mayans R, Keyes JW, et al. SPRINT: A stationary detector single photon ring tomograph for brain imaging. IEEE Transactions on Medical Imaging. 1982;**1**(1):63-68

[14] Rasulo F, Matta B, Varanini N. Cerebral Blood Flow Monitoring. In: Prabhakar H, editor. Neuromonitoring Techniques [Internet]. London, UK: Academic Press; 2018 [cited 2021 Dec

14]. pp. 31-56. Available from: https://linkinghub.elsevier.com/retrieve/pii/B9780128099155000024

[15] Nemoto H, Nakai Y, Hatakeyama R, Shikano N, Jesmin S, Yamaguchi N. Measurement of cerebral blood flow with 99mTc-ECD SPECT and its potential clinical implications--analyzing the relationships between CBF and lifestyle disease. Kaku Igaku. 2012;**49**(4):329-340

[16] Bailey DL, Willowson KP. Quantitative SPECT/CT: SPECT joins PET as a quantitative imaging modality. European Journal of Nuclear Medicine and Molecular Imaging. 2014;**41**(S1):17-25

[17] Jadvar H, Strauss HW, Segall GM. SPECT and PET in the evaluation of coronary artery disease. Radiographics. 1999;**19**(4):915-926

[18] Yonas H, Pindazola RR, Johnson DW. Xenon/computed tomography cerebral blood flow and its use in clinical management. Neurosurgery Clinics of North America. 1996;**7**(4):605-616

[19] Pindzola RR, Yonas H. The xenon-enhanced computed tomography cerebral blood flow method. Neurosurgery. 1998;**43**(6):1488-1491

[20] Massaro LM. Xenon-enhanced CT: Clinical applications. The Journal of Cardiovascular Nursing. 1998;**13**(1):44-56

[21] Carlson AP, Brown AM, Zager E, Uchino K, Marks MP, Robertson C, et al. Xenon-enhanced cerebral blood flow at 28% xenon provides uniquely safe access to quantitative, clinically useful cerebral blood flow information: A multicenter study. AJNR: American Journal of Neuroradiology. 2011;**32**(7):1315-1320

[22] Petcharunpaisan S, Ramalho J, Castillo M. Arterial spin labeling in neuroimaging. World Journal of Radiology. 2010;**2**(10):384-398

[23] Williams DS, Detre JA, Leigh JS, Koretsky AP. Magnetic resonance imaging of perfusion using spin inversion of arterial water. Proceedings of the National Academy of Sciences. 1992;**89**(1):212-216

[24] Detre JA, Zhang W, Roberts DA, Silva AC, Williams DS, Grandis DJ, et al. Tissue specific perfusion imaging using arterial spin labeling. NMR in Biomedicine. 1994;**7**(1-2):75-82

[25] Petersen ET, Lim T, Golay X. Model-free arterial spin labeling quantification approach for perfusion MRI. Magnetic Resonance in Medicine. 2006;**55**(2):219-232

[26] Wolf RL, Detre JA. Clinical neuroimaging using arterial spin-labeled perfusion magnetic resonance imaging. Neurotherapeutics. 2007;**4**(3):346-349

[27] Wu B, Wang X, Guo J, Xie S, Wong EC, Zhang J, et al. Collateral circulation imaging: MR perfusion territory arterial spin-labeling at 3T. AJNR: American Journal of Neuroradiology. 2008;**29**(10):1855-1860

[28] van Laar PJ, van der Grond J, Hendrikse J. Brain perfusion territory imaging: Methods and clinical applications of selective arterial spin-labeling MR imaging. Radiology. 2008;**246**(2):354-364

[29] Paiva FF, Tannús A, Silva AC. Measurement of cerebral perfusion territories using arterial spin labelling. NMR in Biomedicine. 2007;**20**(7):633-642

[30] Golay X, Hendrikse J, Lim TCC. Perfusion imaging using arterial spin labeling. Topics in Magnetic Resonance Imaging: TMRI. 2004;**15**(1):10-27

[31] Detre JA, Alsop DC, Vives LR, Maccotta L, Teener JW, Raps EC. Noninvasive MRI evaluation of cerebral blood flow in cerebrovascular disease. Neurology. 1998;**50**(3):633-641

[32] Chen J, Licht DJ, Smith SE, Agner SC, Mason S, Wang S, et al. Arterial spin labeling perfusion MRI in pediatric arterial ischemic stroke: Initial experiences. Journal of Magnetic Resonance Imaging. 2009;**29**(2):282-290

[33] Du AT, Jahng GH, Hayasaka S, Kramer JH, Rosen HJ, Gorno-Tempini ML, et al. Hypoperfusion in frontotemporal dementia and Alzheimer disease by arterial spin labeling MRI. Neurology. 2006;**67**(7):1215-1220

[34] Sandson TA, O'Connor M, Sperling RA, Edelman RR, Warach S. Noninvasive perfusion MRI in Alzheimer's disease. Neurology. 1996;**47**(5):1339-1342

[35] Engelhorn T, Doerfler A, Weise J, Baehr M, Forsting M, Hufnagel A. Cerebral perfusion alterations during the acute phase of experimental generalized status epilepticus: Prediction of survival by using perfusion-weighted MR imaging and histopathology. AJNR: American Journal of Neuroradiology. 2005;**26**(6):1563-1570

[36] Pollock JM, Tan H, Kraft RA, Whitlow CT, Burdette JH, Maldjian JA. Arterial spin-labeled MR perfusion imaging: Clinical applications. Magnetic Resonance Imaging Clinics of North America. 2009;**17**(2):315-338

[37] Lohrke J, Frenzel T, Endrikat J, Alves FC, Grist TM, Law M, et al. 25 years of contrast-enhanced MRI: Developments, current challenges and future perspectives. Advances in Therapy. 2016;**33**(1):1-28

[38] Young IR, Clarke GJ, Baffles DR, Pennock JM, Doyle FH, Bydder GM. Enhancement of relaxation rate with paramagnetic contrast agents in NMR imaging. Journal of Computed Tomography. 1981;**5**(6):543-547

[39] Xiao YD, Paudel R, Liu J, Ma C, Zhang ZS, Zhou SK. MRI contrast agents: Classification and application (review). International Journal of Molecular Medicine. 2016;**38**(5):1319-1326

[40] Lin YJ, Koretsky AP. Manganese ion enhances T1-weighted MRI during brain activation: An approach to direct imaging of brain function. Magnetic Resonance in Medicine. 1997;**38**(3):378-388

[41] Marckmann P, Skov L, Rossen K, Dupont A, Damholt MB, Heaf JG, et al. Nephrogenic systemic fibrosis: Suspected causative role of gadodiamide used for contrast-enhanced magnetic resonance imaging. Journal of the American Society of Nephrology. 2006;**17**(9):2359-2362

[42] Lee H, Shahrivarkevishahi A, Lumata JL, Luzuriaga MA, Hagge LM, Benjamin CE, et al. Supramolecular and biomacromolecular enhancement of metal-free magnetic resonance imaging contrast agents. Chemical Science. 2020;**11**(8):2045-2050

[43] Korhonen V, Myllylä T, Kirillin MY, Popov AP, Bykov AV, Gorshkov AV, et al. Light propagation in NIR spectroscopy of the human brain. IEEE Journal of Selected Topics in Quantum Electronics. 2014;**20**(2):1-10

[44] Myllylä T, Harju M, Korhonen V, Bykov A, Kiviniemi V, Meglinski I. Assessment of the dynamics of human glymphatic system by near-infrared spectroscopy. Journal of Biophotonics. 2018;**11**(8):e201700123. DOI: 10.1002/jbio.201700123

[45] Eke A, Hermán P, Hajnal M. Fractal and noisy CBV dynamics in humans: Influence of age and gender. Journal of Cerebral Blood Flow and Metabolism. 2006;**26**(7):891-898

[46] Kusaka T, Isobe K, Yasuda S, Koyano K, Nakamura S, Nakamura M, et al. Evaluation of cerebral circulation and oxygen metabolism in infants using near-infrared light. Brain and Development. 2014;**36**(4):277-283

[47] Kay VL, Rickards CA. The role of cerebral oxygenation and regional cerebral blood flow on tolerance to central hypovolemia. American Journal of Physiology-Regulatory, Integrative and Comparative Physiology. 2016;**310**(4):R375-R383

[48] Zaproudina N, Rissanen APE, Lipponen JA, Vierola A, Rissanen SM, Karjalainen PA, et al. Tooth clenching induces abnormal cerebrovascular responses in migraineurs. Frontiers in Neurology. 2018;**9**:1-8

[49] Yagi T, Nagao K, Sakatani K, Kawamorita T, Soga T, Kikushima K, et al. changes of cerebral oxygen metabolism and hemodynamics during ecpr with hypothermia measured by near-infrared spectroscopy: A pilot study. Advances in Experimental Medicine and Biology. 2013;**789**: 121-128

[50] Jelfs B, Banaji M, Tachtsidis I, Cooper CE, Elwell CE. Modelling Noninvasively Measured Cerebral Signals during a Hypoxemia Challenge: Steps towards Individualised Modelling. PLoS One. 2012;**7**(6):e38297

[51] Karthikeyan P, Moradi S, Ferdinando H, Zhao Z, Myllylä T. Optics based label-free techniques and applications in brain monitoring. Applied Sciences. 2020;**10**(6):2196

[52] Igarashi T, Sakatani K, Fujiwara N, Murata Y, Suma T, Shibuya T, et al. Monitoring of hemodynamic change in patients with carotid artery stenosis during the tilt test using wearable near-infrared spectroscopy. In: Van Huffel S, Naulaers G, Caicedo A, Bruley DF, Harrison DK, editors. Oxygen Transport to Tissue XXXV. Advances in Experimental Medicine and Biology, vol 789. New York, NY: Springer; 2013. pp. 463-467. DOI: 10.1007/978-1-4614-7411-1_62

[53] Selb J, Boas DA, Chan S-T, Evans KC, Buckley EM, Carp SA. Sensitivity of near-infrared spectroscopy and diffuse correlation spectroscopy to brain hemodynamics: Simulations and experimental findings during hypercapnia. Neurophotonics. 2014;**1**(1):015005

[54] Boas DA, Sakadžic S, Selb J, Farzam P, Angela Franceschini M, Carp SA. Establishing the diffuse correlation spectroscopy signal relationship with blood flow. Neurophotonics. 2016;**3**(3):031412

[55] Khalid M, Khalid M, Milej D, Milej D, Rajaram A, Rajaram A, et al. Development of a stand-alone DCS system for monitoring absolute cerebral blood flow. Biomedical Optics Express. 2019;**10**(9):4607-4620

[56] Durduran T, Yodh AG. Diffuse correlation spectroscopy for non-invasive, micro-vascular cerebral blood flow measurement. NeuroImage. 2014;**85**:51-63

[57] Selb J, Wu K-C, Sutin J, Lin P-YI, Farzam P, Bechek S, et al. Prolonged monitoring of cerebral blood flow and autoregulation with diffuse correlation spectroscopy in neurocritical care patients. Neurophotonics. 2018;**5**(4):045005

[58] Ferradal SL, Yuki K, Vyas R, Ha CG, Yi F, Stopp C, et al. Non-invasive

assessment of cerebral blood flow and oxygen metabolism in neonates during hypothermic cardiopulmonary bypass: Feasibility and clinical implications. Scientific Reports. 2017;**7**(1):44117

[59] Ferrari M, Quaresima V. The future of noninvasive neonatal brain assessment: The measure of cerebral blood flow by diffuse correlation spectroscopy in combination with near-infrared spectroscopy oximetry. Journal of Perinatology. 2021;**41**(11):2690-2691

[60] Tamborini D, Stephens KA, Wu MM, Farzam P, Siegel AM, Shatrovoy O, et al. Portable system for time-domain diffuse correlation spectroscopy. IEEE Transactions on Biomedical Engineering. 2019;**66**(11):3014-3025

[61] Milej D, Shahid M, Abdalmalak A, Rajaram A, Diop M, St. Lawrence K. Characterizing dynamic cerebral vascular reactivity using a hybrid system combining time-resolved near-infrared and diffuse correlation spectroscopy. Biomedical Optics Express. 2020;**11**(8):4571-4585

[62] Aaslid R, Markwalder TM, Nornes H. Noninvasive transcranial Doppler ultrasound recording of flow velocity in basal cerebral arteries. Journal of Neurosurgery. 1982;**57**(6):769-774

[63] Viski S, Olah L. Use of transcranial Doppler in intensive care unit. Journal of Critical Care Medicine (Universitatea de Medicina si Farmacie din Targu-Mures). 2017;**3**(3):99-104

[64] Blanco P, Abdo-Cuza A. Transcranial Doppler ultrasound in neurocritical care. Journal of Ultrasound. 2018;**21**(1):1-16

[65] Ali MFA. Transcranial Doppler ultrasonography (uses, limitations, and potentials): A review article. Egyptian Journal of Neurosurgery. 2021;**36**(1):1-9

[66] Lipnick MS, Cahill EA, Feiner JR, Bickler PE. Comparison of transcranial Doppler and ultrasound-tagged near infrared spectroscopy for measuring relative changes in cerebral blood flow in human subjects. Anesthesia & Analgesia. 2018;**126**(2):579-587

[67] Racheli N, Ron A, Metzger Y, Breskin I, Enden G, Balberg M, et al. Non-invasive blood flow measurements using ultrasound modulated diffused light. In: Proc SPIE 8223 Photons plus Ultrasound: Imaging and Sensing; 21-26 January 2012; San Francisco, California, United States: SPIE Press; 2012. p. 822332A

[68] Cardim D, Griesdale DE. Near-infrared spectroscopy: Unfulfilled promises. British Journal of Anaesthesia. 2018;**121**(3):523-526

[69] Alqadami ASM, Zamani A, Trakic A, Abbosh A. Flexible electromagnetic cap for three-dimensional electromagnetic head imaging. IEEE Transactions on Biomedical Engineering. 2021;**68**(9):2880-2891

[70] Tournier P, Bonazzoli M, Dolean V, Rapetti F, Hecht F, Nataf F, et al. Numerical modeling and high-speed parallel computing: New perspectives on tomographic microwave imaging for brain stroke detection and monitoring. IEEE Antennas and Propagation Magazine. 2017;**59**(5):98-110

[71] Särestöniemi M, Pomalaza-Raez C, Hakala J, Myllymäki S, Kilpijärvi J, Iinatti J, et al. Detection of brain hemorrhage in white matter using analysis of radio channel characteristics. In: Alam MM, Hämäläinen M, Mucchi L, Niazi IK, le Moullec Y, editors. Body Area Networks Smart IoT and Big Data for Intelligent Health BODYNETS 2020 Lecture Notes of the Institute for Computer Sciences, Social Informatics

and Telecommunications Engineering. Cham, Switzerland: Springer; 2020. pp. 34-45

[72] Mesri HY. Localization of hemorrhage site in stroke patients using multichannel microwave measurements. In: 2012 Annual International Conference of the IEEE Engineering in Medicine and Biology Society; 28 Aug-1 Sept 2012; San Diego, CA, USA: IEEE; 2012. pp. 5927-5930

[73] Abbosh A. Microwave systems for head imaging: Challenges and recent developments. In: 2013 IEEE MTT-S International Microwave Workshop Series on RF and Wireless Technologies for Biomedical and Healthcare Applications (IMWS-BIO); 9-11 December 2013; Singapore: IEEE; 2013. pp. 1-3

[74] Hakala J, Kilpijarvi J, Sarestoniemi M, Hamalainen M, Myllymaki S, Myllyla T. Microwave sensing of brain water—a simulation and experimental study using human brain models. IEEE Access. 2020;**8**:111303-111315

[75] Hossain A, Islam MT, Islam MS, Chowdhury MEH, Almutairi AF, Razouqi QA, et al. A YOLOv3 deep neural network model to detect brain tumor in portable electromagnetic imaging system. IEEE Access. 2021;**9**:82647-82660

[76] Saleeb DA, Helmy RM, Areed NFF, Marey M, Abdulkawi WM, Elkorany AS. A technique for the early detection of brain cancer using circularly polarized reconfigurable antenna array. IEEE Access. 2021;**9**:133786-133794

[77] Groumpas E, Koutsoupidou M, Karanasiou IS, Papageorgiou C, Uzunoglu N. Real-time passive brain monitoring system using near-field microwave radiometry. IEEE Transactions on Biomedical Engineering. 2020;**67**(1):158-165

[78] Ojaroudi M, Bila S, Leveque P, Carré P. Functional microwave imagining system based on cognitive scanning for brain activities monitoring: A feasibility study. In: 2019 13th European Conference on Antennas and Propagation (EuCAP); 31 March-5 April 2019; Krakow, Poland: IEEE; 2019. pp. 1-5

[79] Ojaroudi M, Bila S. Dynamic short-range sensing approach using MIMO radar for brain activities monitoring. In: 2020 14th European Conference on Antennas and Propagation (EuCAP); 15-20 March 2020; Copenhagen, Denmark: IEEE; 2020. pp. 1-5

[80] Ojaroudi M, Bila S. Multiple time-variant targets detection using MIMO radar framework for cerebrovascular monitoring. In: 2021 15th European Conference on Antennas and Propagation (EuCAP); 22-26 March 2021; Dusseldorf, Germany: IEEE; 2021. pp. 1-5

[81] Lauteslager T, Nicolaou N, Lande TS, Constandinou T. Functional neuroimaging using UWB impulse radar: A feasibility study. In: 2015 IEEE Biomedical Circuits and Systems Conference (BioCAS); 22-24 Oct 2015; Atlanta, GA, USA: IEEE; 2015. pp. 1-4

[82] Karanasiou IS, Uzunoglu NK, Papageorgiou CC. Towards functional noninvasive imaging of excitable tissues inside the human body using focused microwave radiometry. IEEE Transactions on Microwave Theory and Techniques. 2004;**52**(8):1898-1908

[83] Maccarini PF, Shah A, Palani SY, Pearce DV, Vardhan M, Stauffer PR, et al. A novel compact microwave radiometric sensor to noninvasively track deep tissue thermal profiles. In: 2015 European

Microwave Conference (EuMC); 7-10 September 2015; Paris, France: IEEE; 2015. pp. 690-693

[84] Momenroodaki P, Haines W, Fromandi M, Popovic Z. Noninvasive internal body temperature tracking with near-field microwave radiometry. IEEE Transactions on Microwave Theory and Techniques. 2018;**66**(5):2535-2545

[85] Tofighi M, Huynh CT. A microwave system for blood perfusion measurements of tissue; a preliminary study. In: 2013 IEEE Topical Conference on Biomedical Wireless Technologies, Networks, and Sensing Systems; 20-23 Jan 2013; Austin, TX, USA: IEEE; 2013. pp. 49-51

[86] Stauffer PR, Snow BW, Rodrigues DB, Salahi S, Oliveira TR, Reudink D, et al. Non-invasive measurement of brain temperature with microwave radiometry: Demonstration in a head phantom and clinical case. The Neuroradiology Journal. 2014;**27**(1):3-12

[87] Karathanasis KT, Gouzouasis IA, Karanasiou IS, Uzunoglu NK. Experimental study of a hybrid microwave radiometry—hyperthermia apparatus with the use of an anatomical head phantom. IEEE Transactions on Information Technology in Biomedicine. 2012;**16**(2):241-247

[88] Karanasiou IS, Uzunoglu NK. Experimental study of 3D contactless conductivity detection using microwave radiometry: A possible method for investigation of brain conductivity fluctuations. In: The 26th Annual International Conference of the IEEE Engineering in Medicine and Biology Society; 1-5 September 2004; San Francisco, CA, USA: IEEE; 2004. pp. 2303-2306

[89] Ojaroudi M, Bila S. Pattern-reconfigurable metasurface-antenna array for functional brain imaging applications. In: 2021 15th European Conference on Antennas and Propagation (EuCAP); 22-26 March 2021; Dusseldorf, Germany: IEEE; 2021. pp. 1-5

[90] Myllylä T, Toronov V, Claassen J, Kiviniemi V, Tuchin V. Near-infrared spectroscopy in multimodal brain research. In: Tuchin V, editor. Handbook of Optical Biomedical Diagnostics. 2nd ed. Vol. 1: Light-Tissue Interaction. Bellingham, Washington, USA: SPIE PRESS; 2016

[91] Myllylä T, Korhonen V, Vihriälä E, Sorvoja H, Hiltunen T, Tervonen O, et al. Human heart pulse wave responses measured simultaneously at several sensor placements by two MR-compatible fibre optic methods. Journal of Sensors. 2012;**2012**:1-9

[92] Myllylä T, Zacharias N, Korhonen V, Zienkiewicz A, Hinrichs H, Kiviniemi V, et al. Multimodal brain imaging with magnetoencephalography: A method for measuring blood pressure and cardiorespiratory oscillations. Scientific Reports. 2017;**7**(1):1-9

[93] Rostrup E, Law I, Pott F, Ide K, Knudsen GM. Cerebral hemodynamics measured with simultaneous PET and near-infrared spectroscopy in humans. Brain Research. 2002;**954**(2):183-193

[94] Vasdekis SN, Tsivgoulis G, Athanasiadis D, Andrikopoulou A, Voumvourakis K, Lazaris AM, et al. Cerebrovascular reacivity assessment in patients with carotid artery disease: A combined TCD and NIRS study. Journal of Neuroimaging. 2012;**22**(3):261-265

[95] Gavgani AM, Wong RHX, Howe PRC, Hodgson DM, Walker FR, Nalivaiko E. Cybersickness-related changes in brain hemodynamics: A

pilot study comparing transcranial Doppler and near-infrared spectroscopy assessments during a virtual ride on a roller coaster. Physiology & Behavior. 2018;**191**:56-64

[96] Raitamaa L, Korhonen V, Huotari N, Raatikainen V, Hautaniemi T, Kananen J, et al. Breath hold effect on cardiovascular brain pulsations—A multimodal magnetic resonance encephalography study. Journal of Cerebral Blood Flow and Metabolism. 2019;**39**(12):2471-2485

[97] Ren H, Jiang X, Xu K, Chen C, Yuan Y, Dai C, et al. A review of cerebral hemodynamics during sleep using near-infrared spectroscopy. Frontiers in Neurology. 2020;**11**:524009

[98] Furtner M, Staudacher M, Frauscher B, Brandauer E, Esnaola y Rojas MM, Gschliesser V, et al. Cerebral vasoreactivity decreases overnight in severe obstructive sleep apnea syndrome: A study of cerebral hemodynamics. Sleep Medicine. 2009;**10**(8):875-881

[99] Wartenberg KE, Schmidt JM, Mayer SA. Multimodality monitoring in neurocritical care. Critical Care Clinics. 2007;**23**(3):507-538

[100] Glover GH. Overview of functional magnetic resonance imaging. Neurosurgery Clinics of North America. 2011;**22**(2):133-139

[101] Ogawa S, Lee T-M, Stepnoski R, Chen W, Zhu X-H, Ugurbil K. An approach to probe some neural systems interaction by functional MRI at neural time scale down to milliseconds. Proceedings of the National Academy of Sciences. 2000;**97**(20):11026-11031

Section 3

Cerebral Venous Circulation

Chapter 5

The Cerebral Venous System: New Pathophysiological Theories and Diseases Related to Veins Occlusion

Giorgio Mantovani and Alba Scerrati

Abstract

Cerebral physiology and pathology are still frequently missing a comprehensive explanation and a complete description, but new data and hypothesis are emerging on a daily basis. Particularly, comprehension of the cerebral venous system's functions and functioning has undergone through the last decades a deep and extended change. Depiction of the perivascular spaces and the mechanisms of glymphatic system has given light about venous system pivotal role in the genesis of different pathologies such as multiple sclerosis, hydrocephalus, cerebral hemorrhages, and strokes. After a key point discussion about embryology, physiology, and anatomy of the cerebral venous system, an overview is provided on the main pathologies, both well-known and newly described ones, in which cerebral veins act a major pathogenic role.

Keywords: cerebral venous system, glymphatic, multiple sclerosis, cerebral vein thrombosis, eagle jugular syndrome, JEDI syndrome

1. Introduction

The cerebral venous system (CVS) is a wide, dynamic, and connected net of vessels developing from the encephalic parenchyma to the internal jugular veins (IJVs). As other venous system, it has three main functions: to drain blood and catabolites from the brain, to help maintaining thermic homeostasis and to refill the right-sided heart [1]. Differently from other organs, instead, intracranial veins share unique physiological features and functions. Traditionally, comprehension of CVS has been limited to descriptive anatomy and a few ranges of physiological principles.

New emerging evidences in the last years are depicting a more complex scenario, in which CVS has a pivotal role in starting and sustaining various pathological processes, from multiple sclerosis to cerebral hemorrhages, hydrocephalus, and strokes.

2. A look into the normal basic anatomy, physiology, and new theories about the glymphatic system

2.1 Developmental embryology

Primitive CVS starts differentiating from primary meninx mesenchyme as a continuous endothelial plexus connecting the dural (*ectomeninx*, the outer portion of primary meninx) and the pia (*endomeninx*, the inner portion) layers. In the first trimester, around the 12th week, a progressive coalescence and resorption of vessels reduces the dura-pial anastomosis to 10–18 bridging veins with specific anatomical features. On the other side, the ectomeninx form the dural folds (falx and tentorium), containing the progressively forming dural sinuses. This early and definitive separation between the parenchymal and dural CVS gives the basis for the blood-brain barrier (BBB) formation [2].

Classically, first clearly identifiable parenchymal vessels are the prootic, the anterior cerebral, and the capitis lateralis and medialis veins [3].

From the 4th to the 5th months, the cortical veins net rapidly grows to sustain the hemisphere fast development. Consequently, the dural sinuses size increases with multiple series of anatomical variations and modifications from week to week. The transverse sinus balloons in response to this increasing amount of blood and to the relatively narrow diameters of jugular vein, with formation and enlargement of multiple emissary vessels for extracranial drainage to the foramen magnum and vertebral plexuses [4]. At the 35-mm stage of the embryo, drainage from the transverse sinus to the IJV can be detected [4].

After birth to the 1st year, the jugular bulb increases in size thanks to the physiological modifications of postnatal circulation, and the drainage through the emissary veins reduces its flow.

2.2 Basic anatomy

Throughout the uterine life, CVS anatomy is dynamically changing in response to the morphometric and hemodynamic adaptations of the growing organism. Progressively, from the chaotic but not homogenous primitive plexus, certain preferential routes are selected on the basis of rheologic flow parameters, while others disappear. The most suitable venous patterns are fixed, independently from our anatomical classifications, similarly to what happens for arteries but with far more variability.

In the ideal description, CVS can be distinguished in parenchymal and dural circulation. It is important to notice that intracranial veins are lacking of intraluminal valves, differently from other veins in the systemic circulation.

The deep parenchymal circulation drains blood from the deep white matter of the cerebral hemisphere, the basal ganglia, and the mesencephalon.

Dural CVS is comprised into the dural sinuses, spaces originated from the splitting of the dura derived from the ectomeninx and covered by endothelium, as above specified.

2.3 Physiology

Arterial blood enters the brain through the anterior circulation, via the carotid arteries, and the posterior circulation, via the vertebral arteries. Also venous blood, or at least the major part of it, exits the brain through an anterior circulation, via the IJVs, and a posterior one, via the vertebral plexuses. Once passed the osteo-dural ring of their respective entry points inside the skull, circulatory physiology of these vessels drastically changes, given the unique physical conditions that are present in the intracranial space.

Although an exhaustive dissertation on cerebrovascular physiology is not in the focus of the present chapter; to understand CVS physiology, few mechanical, hydrostatic, and anatomical principles have to be clarified.

The skull (bone and dura together) is basically a rigid, non-expandable container, totally filled with uncompressible materials: brain parenchyma, blood and cerebrospinal fluid (CSF).

Around 1764, Alexander Monro, second of his name, published *Observations on the Structure and Functions of the Nervous System* [5], in which he theorized his famous principle: "*For, as the substance of the brain, like that of the other solids of our body, is nearly incompressible, the quantity of blood within the head must be the same, or very nearly the same, at all times, whether in health or disease, in life or after death*" [5]. Few years later, George Kellie, one of his students, and John Abercrombie, a pathologist, confirmed his findings and endorsed his theory.

In 1926, Harvey Cushing published "*Studies in intracranial physiology & surgery; the third circulation, the hypophysics, the gliomas*" [6] in which he summarized previous knowledge about intracranial physiology. One of the results of this milestone book was the easy-to-remember equation about Monro-Kellie principle:

$$\text{Brain volume} + \text{CSF} + \text{blood } vol = \text{K} \tag{1}$$

This is an effective way to summarize the concept, but this formulation lacks the fundamental pulsating nature of cerebral flow. Blood enters the brain pulsating in the arteries; then the mechanical wave of pulsation is transmitted anisotropically through the parenchyma and CSF (fluids with different elastic properties). This wave propagation deeply affects CVS physiology: if blood enters the skull pulsating into the arteries, also it leaves from the vein pulsating.

In this balance of pressure between inflow and outflow, bridging veins have a pivotal role.

A bridging vein is defined as a cortical vessel that drains venous blood from the parenchyma to the sinuses, detaching from the cortex and crossing the subarachnoidal CSF filled and the subdural space. It has thin walls (subdural portion 10–600 μm; subarachnoid space of 50–200 μm) with loose collagen network and no muscular fibers [7]. So constituted, it acts as a perfect Starling resistor: a collapsible tube, filled with a fluid exerting pressure (P1, blood venous pressure), inside a space filled with another fluid exerting a different pressure (P2, CSF/intracranial pressure). To maintain a flow inside the tube, it is necessary that P1 > P2.

While entering, or exiting, the cerebral cortex, the superficial arteries and veins in the subarachnoid space are ensheathed in a leptomeningeal coverage, filled with CSF in a double triangle shape. These invaginations are known as Virchow-Robin spaces in their original description [8] and previously taught to be a virtual space, enlarged only in pathological processes. Further studies during the last decades reassessed the importance of these channels and prosecuted their anatomical micro description, thus renaming it perivascular spaces (PVSs).

Deeper into the parenchyma, PVS surrounds the penetrating arteries and capillaries, and it includes a real space that exists between the endothelial basement membrane (aka *basal lamina*), a thin lamina of extracellular matrix components, and *glia limitans*, defined as the barrier formed by perivascular end feet of astrocytes, rich in channel proteins as aquaporin-4 (AQP4) [9]. At the same time, vascular endothelial cells are linked each other by tight junctions, one of the main components of blood-brain barrier (BBB) that restrict macromolecules diffusion inside the parenchyma.

This anatomical description is better defined for the arterial side of cerebral circulation, while venous PVS has not been thoroughly characterized yet.

Intracranial fluids can be divided in intracellular fluid (ICF, 60–70%), interstitial or extracellular fluid (ISF 20% 280–300 mL), blood (10%), and CSF (10% 140–150 mL). Passage of ions, solutes, and molecules between one compartment and the others is precisely regulated to maintain the different chemical composition necessary to their respective physiological role (e.g. plasma contains approximately 270 times more proteins than ISF) [10].

2.4 Glymphatic system

From 2012, a series of experiment on animals and mathematical models led to the discovery and description of the so-called "*glymphatic system*" [11]. This physiological mechanism is taught to act as a cerebral lymphatic system, seen that cerebral tissues lacks a properly formed net of lymphatic vessels and nodes. It is proposed that water from the CSF enters the interstitium by the PVS of the penetrating vessels and capillaries, passing through the filtering glia limitans. Even if the fluid production per capillaries may be too little to be detectable, the total volume of fluid generated by the whole capillary endothelium (an estimated a 20 m^2 surface [9]) is quite considerable. Once interstitial, this water convectively flushes solutes and waste products, such as amyloid β oligomers, into the paravenous CSF space to be discharged.

The first evidence of an intraparenchymal bulk flow along PVS was provided by Cserr [12] in 1974 by following injected tracers.

Fluid exchanges between venular lumen and paravascular space depend primarily on transmural pressure (TMP), a fundamental hemodynamic parameter. Considering the venous wall as the exchange border for fluids, TMP is a differential pressure between internal (intravenous) pressure (IP) and external (paravascular) pressure (EP). EP is represented by the oncotic pressure of the interstitium plus the intracranial pressure (ICP). IP is the sum of blood pressure and the relative venous oncotic pressure. In turn, each of these parameters depends on several others. Of main interest is that venous pressure of parenchymal vessels depends on bridging veins (Starling resistors) function. To sustain a reabsorption flow from the parenchyma to the CVS, it is necessary that IP is lower than EP.

So, in this paradigm, a dynamic balance between CSF, ICF, ISF, and blood is continuously rearranged throughout the entire vascular, arachnoidal, and ependymal surface to maintain the physiological functions of the estimated 16–30 billion neurons of the brain.

Main driving force of this interstitial convective process is the arterial pulsation of the penetrating arteries, moving actively the CSF along the PVS [9]. Alongside, the periodical variation in ICP is generated by breathing (and similar activities that modify intrathoracic pressure) and vasomotor variations in the vascular net.

Glymphatic system function, defined as the capability of flushes toxic solutes away from the parenchyma, normally decline with aging, both in animals and humans. Proposed mechanism is a reduced CSF interstitial influx secondary to decreased pulsatility of sclerotic arteries, impaired CSF production, and reduced AQP4 expression on astrocytes end feet[9]. Hypertension and diabetes mellitus type 2 have also been associated with a decreased glymphatic function. Similar observations have been made in cases of stroke, subarachnoid hemorrhage, traumatic brain injury, and demyelination of various origins.

3. Cerebral vein thrombosis: causes, diagnosis, and treatment

3.1 Clinical presentation

Cerebral vein thrombosis is defined as the presence, in both the cortical vessels and the dural sinuses, of clotted blood impairing physiological flow.

CVT is an uncommon form of stroke (0.5–1% of total), usually affecting young individuals with several associated risk factors (mainly related to Virchow's triad of blood stasis):

- Thrombophilia
- Inflammatory bowel disease
- **Pregnancy** (but als **postpartum** period)
- Dehydration
- Oral contraceptives
- Substance abuse
- **Rheumatologic disorders** (as systemic lupus erythematosus, Behçet disease, sarcoidosis and antiphospholipid and anticardiolipin antibodies)
- **Head trauma** [13].

Other more specific associations are made with:

- **Parameningeal infections** (ear, sinus, mouth, face, and neck)
- Complication of epidural blood patch
- Spontaneous intracranial hypotension
- Lumbar puncture
- **Cancer** (particularly in patients with hematologic malignancies)
- **SARS-CoV2 infection (COVID-19)** [14]
- **Climatic conditions** (particularly high ambient temperatures) [15].

An underestimated risk factor for CVT is a JV thrombosis that propagates cranially, often because of the presence of medical dispositive [13].

Exact epidemiology of CVT is unknown because clinical features are quite variable, and for this reason, cases should be classified differently [16].

Recently, cerebral venous sinus thrombosis in association with COVID-19 has been described, both as a first clinical presentation or a subsequent complication [17].

Clinical findings are related to intracranial hypertension, related to impaired venous drainage, and/or to focal brain injury from venous ischemia or hemorrhage. Obviously, clinical manifestations of CVT also depend on the location of the thrombosis.

Most frequent symptoms are

- **Headache** (90% of patients): typically described as diffuse and often progressive over days to weeks. Less frequently, it may present with thunderclap headache, similar to a subarachnoid hemorrhage, or a migraines-like headache. Up to 25% of patients with CVT only present with headache [16].

- **Seizures** (40% of patients): first, focal, or generalized seizures are frequent.

- **Papilledema or diplopia** (caused by sixth nerve palsy).

- **Neurological signs and deficits**: most common are hemiparesis and aphasia.

- **Scalp edema and dilated scalp veins** may be seen on examination.

When CVT is secondary to regional infection, signs and symptom of the primary cause can be detected: toothache and odontogenic abscess; ear discharge; pain in the ear, face, or mastoid region.

3.2 Laboratory exams

In patients with suspected CVT routine, laboratory essay including complete blood count, chemistry panel, prothrombin time, and activated partial thromboplastin time should be performed [9] in order to identify pro-coagulative systemic status. D-dimer assessment makes sense in presence of low pretest probability of CVT to exclude the diagnosis, similarly to pulmonary embolism. Lumbar puncture is characterized by a high opening pressure (80% of cases) but has limited diagnostic value. It is not routinely indicated unless CNS infection is suspected.

3.3 Red flags to avoid misdiagnosis

Thirty to forty percent of patients with CVT present with an intracranial hemorrhage [18]. Progressively increasing headache over days and alterations in laboratory exams with evidence of hypercoagulability should prompt further radiological assessment for evaluating CVT. Also, at the CT exam, an ischemic/hemorragic lesion that crosses normal arterial boundaries, deep bilateral, or in close proximity to a venous sinus is suggestive of CVT.

Patients complaining of isolated headache and signs or symptoms of intracranial hypertension (papilledema or sixth nerve palsies) should be evaluated for CVT. The correct differential diagnosis between idiopathic intracranial hypertension (IIH) and CVT has therapeutic and prognostic importance. In both cases, however, clinical manifestations are related to the impaired venous outflow function, with subsequent increasing of the ISF.

DOI: http://dx.doi.org/10.5772/intechopen.102351

3.4 Radiological diagnosis

3.4.1 CT scan

In a contest of a CVT suspect case, CT without contrast may demonstrate some characteristic features, but an exact diagnosis is made complex by the intrinsic anatomic variability of the venous sinuses and cortical veins. In fact, only in 30% of CVT cases, CT scan shows some abnormalities [19].

The fundamental sign of acute CVT on a CT (without contrast) is a homogenous hyperdensity of a cortical vein or sinus. Another typical sign of the superior sagittal sinus thrombosis (posterior portion) is the filled delta sign, a dense triangle in the context of the sinus.

Only 0.5–0.8% of patients with CVT showed some signs of subarachnoid hemorrhage, often in atypical position.

The contrast-enhancing CT scan could add some clues, such as the classic "empty delta" sign: an enhancement of the dural border of the sinus with a filling defect within it due to the thrombus in a triangular shape.

This is not a precocious finding, but usually lasts for several weeks after the acute phase.

On the other hand, CT venography is much more useful in chronic follow-up because the occluded sinus cavity shows a variable density. The presence of cortical bone close to the dural sinus can produce interfering artifacts during the visualization of the enhanced dural sinus.

3.4.2 Magnetic resonance imaging

Classically inside the normal sinus, there is a flow void signal due to the venous stream continuously moving. Early signs of CVT can be visualized as *absence* of this flow void with T2 hypointensity or a central iso-hypodense lesion with surrounding enhancement.

Meanwhile, an acute thrombus, not fully formed yet, may appear as a hypointense signal, similar to the normal flow void.

Other signs include cerebral swelling, edema, and/or hemorrhage. Diffusion-weighted imaging (DWI) sequences show hyperintense signal, meaning a reduced blood flow, with a prognostic significance: brightening sinus on DWI predict low chances of recanalization.

Magnetic resonance imaging (MRI) is particularly helpful in defining the nature and extension of parenchymal lesions, causes, or consequences of the CVT: focal edema, infarction, and infectious processes.

MRI venography is the most common CVT diagnostic technique with the use of two-dimensional time-of-flight (TOF) sequences because of its excellent sensitivity to slow flow inside the sinus.

3.4.3 Cerebral angiography

Venous phase of cerebral angiography (4–8 s from the injections) typically, and directly, shows a filling defect in the occluded lumen. Other signs are venous congestion with dilated cortical, scalp, or facial veins, enlargement of collateral drainage, and venous flow reversal.

Although it is an invasive procedure, cerebral angiography (or venography) could help to solve undefined situations due to anatomic variations such as sinus atresia/hypoplasia, asymmetrical drainage, and normal sinus filling defects caused by arachnoid granulations or septa.

3.5 Treatment

Most used therapeutic approach is based on blood anticoagulation, which aims to prevent thrombus growth, avoids development of pulmonary embolism, and promotes sinus recanalization. Different drugs and different strategies are present in literature [16], with the use of unfractionated heparin (UFH), antivitamin K molecules, low-molecular-weight heparin (LMWH), and low-dose unfractionated heparin. An effective treatment is complicated by the presence of intracranial hemorrhage or cerebral infarction at the time of the diagnosis, given the increased risk of worsening the bleeding.

The available data from RCT comparing clinical/radiological outcomes and bleeding complications support a safe and effective role for anticoagulation in the treatment of CVT, even if intracranial bleeding is present [16]. There are no data that suggest the preferential use of UFH or LMWH in CVT patients. Some data suggest that, if pulmonary embolism or deep vein thrombosis is present, LMWH have to be preferred [20].

In case of secondary CVT (infection, trauma, and other transient causes) vitamin-k antagonist should be continued for 6 months after the removal of the causative factor [16].

Otherwise, in case of primary CVT, vitamin-k antagonist should be continued for 6–12 months and further coagulative assessment should be carried on [16].

Other therapeutic options include

- **Fibrinolytic therapy**: preferentially used when clinical worsening is present even if anticoagulation is well conducted, or in case of intracranial hypertension not responsive to other treatments. There are few evidences that fibrinolysis increase the recanalization rate of the occluded sinuses [18]. It could be delivered as systemic therapy or by direct sinus catheterization (thrombolysis), in this case a mechanical thrombectomy can be associated.

- **Surgery**: decompressive craniectomy or hematoma evacuation may be a necessary life-saving measure if a significant increase in intracranial pressure progresses despite conservative treatment.

- **Antibiotics**: mandatory if CVT is secondary to propagating infections, when possible, in association with drainage of purulent sources (subdural empyemas or purulent collections within the paranasal sinuses).

- **Antiepileptic drugs**: indicated only in case of seizures (even one), without preferred molecules, to reduce the risk of anoxic damage.

- **Corticosteroid**: even if useful to reduce vasogenic edema, steroid could alter blood homeostasis and enhance clot formation. There are evidences that steroid increase the overall risk of death or dependence with steroid treatment at 6 months in CVT patients [21].

4. Jugular vein stenosis

Cerebrospinal venous insufficiency is an emerging nosological entity collecting different conditions that shares an impaired venous outflow from the brain to the heart. Multiple central nervous system disorders, such as idiopathic intracranial hypertension (IIH), Ménière disease, transient monocular blindness, and Alzheimer's disease, have already been reported to be associated with internal jugular vein (IJV) stenosis [22, 23]. Nowadays, different branches of medical sciences are directing their attention to the delicate balance between cerebral inflow and outflow in order to better understand CVS physiology and its correlation with several disorders. As a mechanical system, a CVS flow obstruction from any causes at any level lead to an increased pressure transmitted upward. This means an increased capillary pressure, thus an increased TMP and finally a decreased glymphatic paravascular ISF flushing and reabsorption into the CVS. Proceeding from the parenchyma to the major vessels, venous convergence reduces the possibility of alternatively restoring a fully functioning flow. Once in the IJV, collateral drainages are few and of limited caliber. So, at this level, any stenosis (intraluminal, parietal, or extraluminal) produce effects diffused at the entire CVS and to the parenchyma. In the mathematical Gadda-Ursino hemodynamic model of CVS outflow, a jugular stenosis is a significant parameter in sinus pressure regulation [24].

Over the last years, several new pathologies have been described related to IJV obstruction, and old ones received new interpretations.

4.1 JEDI syndrome

Usually, patients suffering from IIH are women with elevated BMI and normal to slit cerebral ventricles [25]. Meanwhile, IIH has a strong relation with impaired CVS outflow caused by increased thoracic-abdominal or dural sinuses pressure (obesity, CVT, and superior vena cava syndrome). On the other hand, acutely dilated ventricles are related to high-pressure hydrocephalus caused by cerebrovascular pathology (infection, trauma, and hemorrhage).

Recently, an anomalous IIH case with dilated ventricle (Evans index 0.36) has been described in a woman with normal BMI complaining of headache, visual loss (Frisen grade 4 papilledema), and pulsating tinnitus. Neuroimaging did not reveal any causes of hydrocephalus from intracranial lesions, while a fluorodeoxyglucose (FDG) positron emission tomography (PET) described a diffuse hypometabolic cerebral state.

At B-mode echography of extracranial IJV, a bilateral external compression from omohyoid muscle was demonstrated, hemodynamically corresponding to blocked venous flow with scarce collateral compensation.

The patient underwent surgical bilateral resection of omohyoid muscle with ICP invasive monitoring. After transection of the muscles, a sudden drop in ICP and normalization of ICP wave were observed.

Headache and tinnitus disappeared after surgery, and papilledema progressively improved with visual acuity restoration. Serial (24 months' follow-up) MRI documented regression of Evans index and FDG-PET showed improvement of brain metabolism.

These peculiar cases led to the description of a new clinical entity, a form of hydrocephalus that does not require CSF shunt procedures. This syndrome has been called JEDI (jugular entrapment dilated ventricles intracranial hypertension) syndrome [26].

While an extracranial obstacle to CVS is coherent with intracranial hypertension for the aforementioned principles, it is still unclear what caused ventricles dilatation in this case. More studies are needed to fully comprehend the relation between IJV obstruction, IIH, and hydrocephalus.

4.2 Eagle jugular syndrome

In 1937, the American otolaryngologist Dr. Eagle was the first to describe a clinical syndrome caused by an elongated styloid process [27]. The stylohyoid complex is composed of styloid process, stylohyoid ligament, and the lesser horn of the hyoid bone. The styloid bone starts from the inferior portion of the temporal bone, just medially to the base of mastoid process, and directs inferiorly, medially, and anteriorly, passing anteriorly and laterally to the C1 anterior arch and transverse process. These anatomical structures embriologically originate from Reichert's cartilage of the second brachial arch.

Classic Eagle syndrome is mainly characterized by pain, dysphagia and otalgia, often exacerbated by yawning and swallowing, arising after a tonsillectomy. It is thought that postsurgical scar tissue stretches the sensory nerves ending in the peripharingeal region [28].

The carotid artery variant of Eagle syndrome is due to the impingement between an elongated styloid process and the carotid artery and associated nerves. It is characterized by pain and an increased risk of cerebrovascular ischemic accidents: arterial dissection, obstruction, transient ischemic attack, and stroke.

A third variant of the syndrome has been described, consisting in an IJV compressed by an elongated styloid process in the passage adjacent to the transverse process of C1. The most common involved jugular segment is J3, and in more than 50% of patients the stenosis is bilateral. It is alternatively named "*Eagle jugular syndrome*," "*Styloidogenic-cervical spondylotic internal jugular venous compression*," or "*Styloid-induced internal jugular vein stenosis*" [29].

This latter form of Eagle syndrome has specific features related to an impaired CVS outflow.

Clinical presentation is frequently nonspecific. Most frequent symptoms are

- **Headache** (46.3%): not typically present in the classic and carotid variant of Eagle syndrome;
- **Tinnitus** (43.6%);
- **Insomnia** (39.6%);
- **Visual disturbances** (28.9%);
- **Hearing impairment** (24.2%).

More peculiar, an **increased ICP** is observed in more than one-third of patients (36.2%).

It is more common in young adults (mean age of onset 38.6 years) with no prevalence between sex.

In literature, only 1/3 of patients with diagnosed Eagle jugular syndrome have an effectively elongated styloid process. This suggests that even with a normal length, an abnormally narrow space between the styloid process and C1 transverse process may lead to IJV compression [30].

Diagnosis is classically radiological, with direct evidence of impaired IJV flow (MRI venography or angiographic venography) or indirect proof of a narrowed C1-styloid space (CT scan or MRI). Few criteria have been proposed, and not diffusely shared between studies, to define a significant IJV stenosis in a setting of suspected Eagle jugular syndrome. According to Jayaraman [31], a jugular stenosis is defined as a caliber reduction >80% on axial cuts compared with the normal vein proximal to the stenosis. Ding and Bai [32] proposed other similar criteria.

More frequently, a conservative treatment is preferred with anticoagulant usage, but in most cases medical therapy has shown no effectiveness on symptoms control.

Invasive procedures are surgical (styloidectomy, C1 anterior arch removal), endovascular (ballooning or stenting), or combination of both. Styloidectomy is the most frequently performed surgical procedure, and major risks are vascular or facial nerve injuries.

On the other side, endovascular treatments are associated with stent migration or fracture, pseudoaneurysm formation, thrombosis, and cranial nerve injuries.

After an invasive approach, more than 70% of patients report an improvement in tinnitus, papilledema, and visual disturbances. Headache, the most frequent symptom, and dizziness usually do not respond to the treatment.

One of the major issues still open regarding the Eagle jugular syndrome is the lack of standardized data, especially on IJV pressure, flow velocity, and collateral pathways. Thus, a complete understanding of pathogenesis is missing.

4.3 Multiple sclerosis

Multiple sclerosis is a complex autoimmune demyelinating disease characterized by a chronic inflammatory response against the CNS. Many aspects of this disease are still unknown, but evidences have increased, through the last decades, pointing toward a fundamental involvement of CVS in the early development of it.

A cardinal observation is that each MS lesion is crossed and split by a central vein, that is to say that demyelination and inflammatory infiltration develop around a vein [33].

From a wider point of view, inflammatory processes in MS seem to be concentrated around venular vessels, more than capillary or arterial [34].

From these data, and others, an association has been proposed between MS and chronic cerebrospinal venous insufficiency (CCSVI), a condition of long-lasting impaired venous drainage from CVS caused by obstruction in extracranial veins. Recently, CCSVI has been associated also with other degenerative processes such as Alzheimer's disease, Parkinson's disease, and Meniere's disease.

A defective valve, hypoplasia, and/or compression of the IJV or the azygos vein, as defined earlier, increase TMP and reduce the ability of glymphatic system to drain toxic catabolites from the interstitium. These peptides then accumulate at the perivenular level and may act as first inflammatory chemotactic activators and further increase oncotic pressure into the perivascular space, worsening the ISF resorption capacity. Generally, perivenular spaces are recognized as an important site of leukocyte trafficking and the potential milestones to modulate immune response.

Measuring CSF dynamic with MRI reveals interesting links between venous function and MS. In clinically isolated syndrome (CIS), conversion to clinically definite MS in the following year has been related to CSF net flow decreasing [35].

In relapsing-remitting MS, a significant reduction in CSF flow at the level of the Sylvius aqueduct was observed compared to control groups [36]. In the early and progressive form of MS, an increase in ventricular dimension has been observed during the first year. This may be related to the impaired function of glymphatic system, and there are evidences that in these patients, a therapeutic flow restoration through endovascular recanalization of IJV is linked to a significant reduction in ventricles and subarachnoid spaces dimension [37].

Moreover, CCSVI is an ultimate cause of decreased cerebral perfusion because of the propagation of retrograde hypertension. There is a linear correlation between flow into the IJV and global brain perfusion [38]. Moreover, in MS, hypoperfusion is a pathological key point that precedes plaque formation and could be a causative agent, provoking damages to the oxygen-dependent oligodendrocytes. Myelin loss and debris occur when the metabolism of these cells is altered, and this is an important inflammatory signal that attracts leukocytes. Thus, inflammation seems to be a consequence, more than a cause [39]. Subsequent BBB disruption causes microbleedings, and iron deposition, coming from hemoglobin degradation, further increases inflammatory response and microbleedings, especially around venular vessels. Consistently, cerebral tissue iron loading correlates with MS-related disability at the Expanded Disability Status Scale (EDSS) [40].

4.4 Perimesencephalic subarachnoidal hemorrhage

A subarachnoidal hemorrhage (SAH) not caused by vascular malformation (such as aneurysm or arteriovenous malformation (AVM) rupture) is a recognized clinical entity usually referred as *sine materia* (without motivations) or non-aneurismatic SAH (na-SAH).

It typically presents with a pattern limited to the perimesencephalic cisterns (typical pattern), sometimes extended to the nearer basal cisterns (atypical pattern). In the majority of cases, the clinical course is benign, with a very low rate of recurrence. At the neuroimaging, no causes of bleeding are detected, neither immediately or later. Pathogenesis of na-SAH is not established, but the most shared hypothesis regards anatomic variations of CVS, particularly of the Basal Vein of Rosenthal (BVR) draining into venous systems different from the Galenic one. CVS hypertension has also been occasionally reported to influence the overall risk of na-SAH in various conditions, such as cavernous sinus thrombosis, transverse sinus thrombosis, or a bilateral jugular venous obstruction.

In a retrospective case-control study, a significant association has been made between na-SAH and the presence of an IJV stenosis (>80% of caliber reduction) at the passage through the styloid process and the arch of C1 [41]. Also, older age and diabetes were statistically linked to an increased risk of na-SAH.

This is coherent with what has been reported before: an impaired CVS outflow due to a stenosis leads to increased venular pressure, thus predisposing wall rupture and bleeding when an adjunctive pressure is applied (e.g. physical exertion). The presence of anatomic variations may be a further element that increases the risk of na-SAH, but, in the end, the way in which venous configuration of the perimesencephalic area might predispose to bleeding remains undetermined.

Author details

Giorgio Mantovani and Alba Scerrati*
University of Ferrara, Ferrara, Italy

*Address all correspondence to: a.scerrati@gmail.com

References

[1] Zamboni P. The contribution of extra cranial venous drainage to neuro-inflammation in multiple sclerosis [Internet]. In: Neuroinflammation. In, Amsterdam, Netherlands: Elsevier; 2018. pp. 579-599. Available from: https://linkinghub.elsevier.com/retrieve/pii/B9780128117095000363

[2] Mack J, Squier W, Eastman JT. Anatomy and development of the meninges: Implications for subdural collections and CSF circulation. Pediatric Radiology. 2009;**39**(3):200-210

[3] Safadi AO, Tadi P. Anatomy, head and neck, cerebral venous system [Internet]. In: StatPearls. Treasure Island (FL): StatPearls Publishing; 2021. Available from: http://www.ncbi.nlm.nih.gov/books/NBK560496/

[4] Okudera T. Development of posterior fossa dural sinuses, emissary veins, and jugular bulb: Morphological and radiologic study. American Journal of Neuroradiology. 1994;**15**:1871-1883

[5] Alexander M. Observations on the Structure and Functions of the Nervous System. Edinburgh; 1783

[6] Cushing H. Studies in Intracranial Physiology & Surgery; the Third Circulation, the Hypophysics, the Gliomas. London: H. Milford, Oxford University Press; 1926

[7] Mortazavi MM, Denning M, Yalcin B, Shoja MM, Loukas M, Tubbs RS. The intracranial bridging veins: A comprehensive review of their history, anatomy, histology, pathology, and neurosurgical implications. Child's Nervous System. 2013;**29**(7):1073-1078

[8] Weed LH. Studies on cerebro-spinal fluid. No. II: The theories of drainage of cerebro-spinal fluid with an analysis of the methods of investigation. The Journal of Medical Research. 1914;**31**(1):21

[9] Klostranec JM, Vucevic D, Bhatia KD, et al. Current concepts in intracranial interstitial fluid transport and the glymphatic system: Part I—Anatomy and physiology. Radiology. 2021;**301**(3):502-514

[10] Hladky SB, Barrand MA. Mechanisms of fluid movement into, through and out of the brain: Evaluation of the evidence. Fluids Barriers CNS. 2014;**11**(1):1-32

[11] Iliff JJ, Wang M, Liao Y, et al. A paravascular pathway facilitates CSF flow through the brain parenchyma and the clearance of interstitial solutes, including amyloid β. Science Translational Medicine. 2012;**4**(147):147ra111-147ra111

[12] Cserr HF, Ostrach LH. Bulk flow of interstitial fluid after intracranial injection of blue dextran 2000. Experimental Neurology. 1974;**45**(1):50-60

[13] Scerrati A, Menegatti E, Zamboni M, et al. Internal jugular vein thrombosis: Etiology, symptomatology, diagnosis and current treatment. Diagnostics. 2021;**11**(2):378

[14] Cavalcanti DD, Raz E, Shapiro M, et al. Cerebral venous thrombosis associated with COVID-19. AJNR. American Journal of Neuroradiology. 2020;**41**(8):1370-1376

[15] Aaron S, Lakshmanan J, Sudarsanam TD, et al. Cerebral venous thrombosis, seasonal trends, and climatic influence: A region-Specific study. Annals of Indian Academy of Neurology. 2020;**23**(4):522-527

[16] Saposnik G, Barinagarrementeria F, Brown RD, et al. Diagnosis and management of cerebral venous thrombosis. Stroke. 2011;**42**(4):1158-1192

[17] Hughes C, Nichols T, Pike M, Subbe C, Elghenzai S. Cerebral venous sinus thrombosis as a presentation of COVID-19. European Journal of Case Reports in Internal Medicine. 2020;7(5):001691

[18] Wasay M, Bakshi R, Bobustuc G, et al. Cerebral venous thrombosis: Analysis of a multicenter cohort from the United States. Journal of Stroke and Cerebrovascular Diseases. 2008;**17**(2): 49-54

[19] Leach JL, Fortuna RB, Jones BV, Gaskill-Shipley MF. Imaging of cerebral venous thrombosis: Current techniques, spectrum of findings, and diagnostic pitfalls. Radiography Review Publishing Radiological Society of North America INC. 2006;**26**(Suppl. 1):S19-41; discussion S42-43

[20] van Dongen CJJ, van den Belt AGM, Prins MH, Lensing AWA. Fixed dose subcutaneous low molecular weight heparins versus adjusted dose unfractionated heparin for venous thromboembolism. Cochrane Database of Systematic Reviews. 2004;**4**:CD001100

[21] Canhão P, Cortesão A, Cabral M, et al. Are steroids useful to treat cerebral venous thrombosis? Stroke. 2008;**39**(1):105-110

[22] Chung C-P, Hsu H-Y, Chao A-C, Sheng W-Y, Soong B-W, Hu H-H. Transient global amnesia: Cerebral venous outflow impairment-insight from the abnormal flow patterns of the internal jugular vein. Ultrasound in Medicine & Biology. 2007;**33**(11):1727-1735

[23] Chung C-P, Beggs C, Wang P-N, et al. Jugular venous reflux and white matter abnormalities in Alzheimer's disease: A pilot study. Journal of Alzheimer's Disease (JAD). 2014;**39**(3):601-609

[24] Gadda G, Taibi A, Sisini F, Gambaccini M, Zamboni P, Ursino M. A new hemodynamic model for the study of cerebral venous outflow. American Journal of Physiology. Heart and Circulatory Physiology. 2015;**308**(3):H217-H231

[25] Mollan SP, Davies B, Silver NC, et al. Idiopathic intracranial hypertension: Consensus guidelines on management. Journal of Neurology, Neurosurgery, and Psychiatry. 2018;**89**(10):1088-1100

[26] De Bonis P, Menegatti E, Cavallo MA, et al. JEDI (jugular entrapment, dilated ventricles, intracranial hypertension) syndrome: A new clinical entity? A case report. Acta Neurochirurgica. 2019;**161**(7):1367-1370

[27] Petrović B, Radak Đ, Kostić V, Čovičković-Šternić N. Styloid syndrome: A review of literature. Srpski Arhiv za Celokupno Lekarstvo. 2008;**136**(11-12):667-674

[28] Fusco DJ, Asteraki S, Spetzler RF. Eagle's syndrome: Embryology, anatomy, and clinical management. Acta Neurochirurgica. 2012;**154**(7):1119-1126

[29] Scerrati A, Norri N, Mongardi L, et al. Styloidogenic-cervical spondylotic internal jugular venous compression, a vascular disease related to several clinical neurological manifestations: Diagnosis and treatment—A comprehensive literature review. Annals of Translational Medicine. 2021;**9**(8):718-718

[30] Ho S, Luginbuhl A, Finden S, Curry JM, Cognetti DM. Styloid/C1 transverse process juxtaposition as a

cause of Eagle's syndrome. Head & Neck. 2015;**37**(11):E153-E156

[31] Jayaraman MV, Boxerman JL, Davis LM, Haas RA, Rogg JM. Incidence of extrinsic compression of the internal jugular vein in unselected patients undergoing CT angiography. AJNR. American Journal of Neuroradiology. 2012;**33**(7):1247-1250

[32] Bai C, Wang Z, Guan J, et al. Clinical characteristics and neuroimaging findings in eagle syndrome induced internal jugular vein stenosis. Annals of Translational Medicine. 2020;**8**(4):97

[33] Sati P, Oh J, Constable RT, et al. The central vein sign and its clinical evaluation for the diagnosis of multiple sclerosis: A consensus statement from the north American imaging in multiple sclerosis cooperative. Nature Reviews. Neurology. 2016;**12**(12):714-722

[34] Ge Y, Zohrabian VM, Grossman RI. Seven-tesla magnetic resonance imaging: New vision of microvascular abnormalities in multiple sclerosis. Archives of Neurology. 2008;**65**(6):812-816

[35] Magnano C, Schirda C, Weinstock-Guttman B, et al. Cine cerebrospinal fluid imaging in multiple sclerosis. Journal of Magnetic Resonance Imaging (JMRI). 2012;**36**(4):825-834

[36] Zamboni P, Menegatti E, Weinstock-Guttman B, et al. The severity of chronic cerebrospinal venous insufficiency in patients with multiple sclerosis is related to altered cerebrospinal fluid dynamics. Functional Neurology. 2009;**24**(3):133-138

[37] Zamboni P, Menegatti E, Cittanti C, et al. Fixing the jugular flow reduces ventricle volume and improves brain perfusion. Journal of Vascular Surgery. Venous and Lymphatic Disorders. 2016;**4**(4):434-445

[38] Utriainen D, Trifan G, Sethi S, et al. Magnetic resonance imaging signatures of vascular pathology in multiple sclerosis. Neurological Research. 2012;**34**(8):780-792

[39] Henderson APD, Barnett MH, Parratt JDE, Prineas JW. Multiple sclerosis: Distribution of inflammatory cells in newly forming lesions. Annals of Neurology. 2009;**66**(6):739-753

[40] Zivadinov R, Heininen-Brown M, Schirda CV, et al. Abnormal subcortical deep-gray matter susceptibility-weighted imaging filtered phase measurements in patients with multiple sclerosis: A case-control study. NeuroImage. 2012;**59**(1):331-339

[41] Scerrati A, De Bonis P, Zamboni P, et al. A new insight in nonaneurysmal subarachnoid hemorrhage: The potential role of the internal jugular veins. Journal of Neurological Surgery Part A: Central European Neurosurgery. 2021;**1**:2. DOI: 10.1055/s-0041-1733895

Chapter 6

Cerebrospinal Venous Obstruction: Anatomy, Clinical Presentation, Diagnosis, and Treatment of Chronic Infective Cerebrospinal Venulitis

Paul K. Thibault

Abstract

This review chapter describes the normal anatomy and function of the cerebrospinal venous system, ultrasound diagnosis of obstructions in the system, and the clinical implications and treatment of chronic cerebrospinal venous obstruction (CCSVO) associated with chronic persistent *Chlamydophila pneumoniae* (*Cpn*) infection. The normal patterns of flow in the cerebrospinal venous system are described and guidelines for the interpretation of the extracranial duplex ultrasound (ECDU) examination of the neck veins are presented. An infective cause of CCSVO is proposed and relevant pathology tests necessary for a diagnosis of chronic persistent *Cpn* venulitis are discussed. A treatment protocol for *Cpn* chronic venulitis is described and recommended. The progress of the patient with CCSVO can then be followed and monitored by using the ECDU and relevant pathology tests after 3 and 6 months. CCSVO is a relatively common condition encountered in chronic diseases of unknown etiology and is often neglected by medical practitioners when managing patients with symptoms of brain fog, chronic headaches, and fatigue. Objective diagnostic and treatment protocols are required to make further progress with these conditions.

Keywords: cerebrospinal venous obstruction, chronic infective venulitis, multiple sclerosis, rosacea, CFS

1. Introduction

The term "cerebrospinal venous system" (CSVS) was first proposed by Tobinik in 2006 to describe the generally valveless venous system that extends from the cranium along the whole length of the spine to the sacrum [1]. In effect the CSVS connects the intracranial veins to the pelvic plexuses and directly or indirectly communicates with organs in the neck, chest, and abdomen. Batson [2], in a series of experiments involving human cadavers and living monkeys, demonstrated the continuity of the CSVS from the cranium to the pelvis and established that the CSVS provided a direct

IntechOpen

vascular route for the spread of tumors, infection, or emboli from the pelvis to the brain. Batson established that the CSVS was primarily valveless thereby allowing venous flow in both directions.

In 1829 Beschet [3] produced detailed drawings depicting the multiple anastomoses of the cranial vertebral veins that led to the recognition of the anatomic and physiologic continuity that exists between the CSVS and the venous sinuses and plexuses of the brain. Groen et al. [4] divided the CSVS into three connecting divisions—the internal vertebral venous plexuses, which surround the spinal cord; the external vertebral venous plexuses (anterior and posterior), which surround the vertebral column; and the basivertebral veins, which run transversely within the vertebrae. The vertebral venous plexuses course longitudinally along the entire length of the spine, from the sacrum to the cranium (**Figure 1**). Groen and colleagues [5] had previously confirmed that all three divisions of the CSVS freely intercommunicate and that all divisions of the CSVS lack valves. The only exception to this is at the cranial end

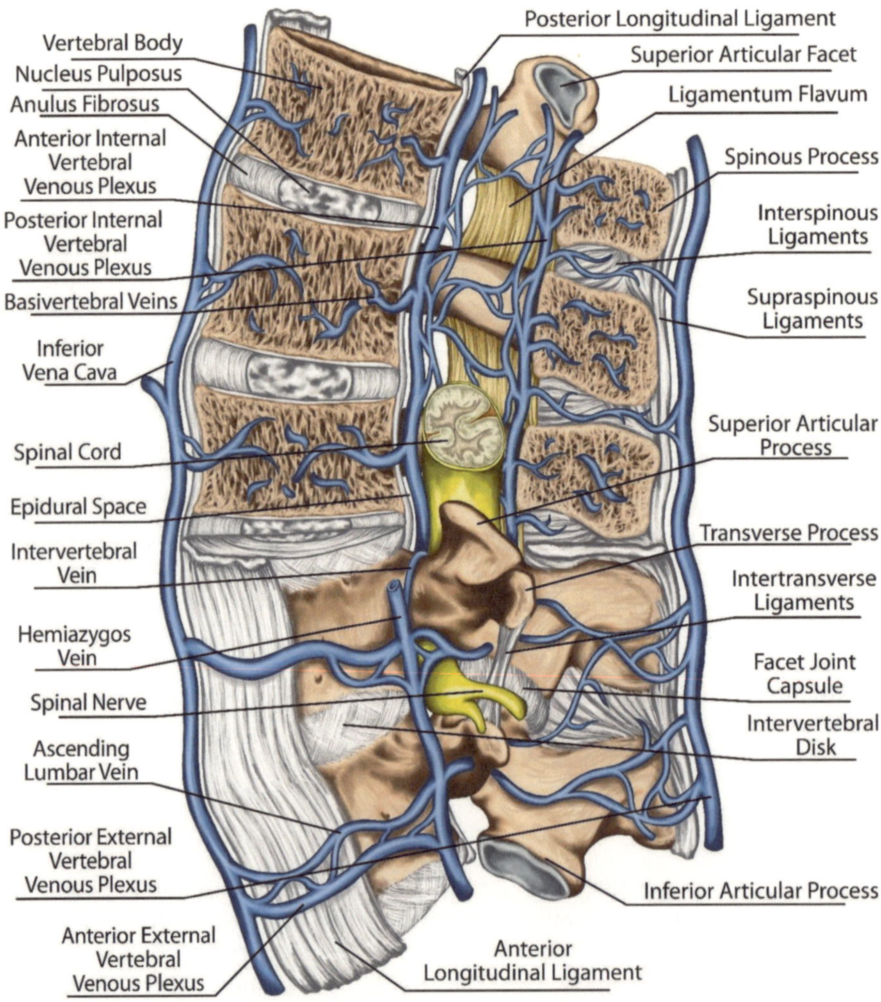

Figure 1.
The vertebral venous plexus comprises an interconnected and richly anastomosed system of veins that run along the entire length of the vertebral column.

where the vertebral veins (VVs) have a terminal valve, where they communicate with brachiocephalic veins in the neck [6].

The anatomic connections between the vertebral venous plexuses and the intracranial venous system have been confirmed by multiple investigators [2–4]. There is also communication among facial veins, ophthalmic and orbital veins, and intracerebral veins [7]. Distally, the CSVS communicates with other superficial valveless veins in the back and thoracoabdominal wall [5, 8]. In addition, the CSVS communicates with the systemic venous system, including the azygous veins (and thereby the posterior bronchial vein and the parietal pleural veins), the left renal and suprarenal veins, the portal venous system, and both vena cava, thereby providing a continuous, bidirectional venous system that both bypasses and communicates with the valve-bearing, directional, systemic venous system [1, 4, 5, 8]. At the caudal end the CSVS freely communicates with the pelvic and prostatic veins and the sacral venous plexus.

2. The normal patterns of flow in the neck veins

A unique feature of cerebral venous drainage is its dependence on posture. While in the supine position the internal jugular veins (IJVs) are the main drainage pathways, in the upright position the IJVs generally collapse with the VVs, internal and external vertebral venous plexuses compensating to a large extent [9–11]. Valdueza et al. [12] using duplex sonography, measured cerebral venous outflow in 23 healthy human volunteers, found that internal jugular flow decreased from 700 mL/minute in the supine position to 70 mL/minute at 90° elevation. They also found a corresponding increase in vertebral vein flow from 40 mL/minute at 0° elevation to 210 mL/min at 90°, with the balance of the unmeasured flow probably passing through the vertebral venous plexuses, which are inaccessible to Doppler measurement. In addition, duplex ultrasound studies have shown that the drainage of the cerebral blood is asymmetric with a preferential outflow via the right IJV and VV [13, 14].

3. Chronic obstruction in the CSVS

Chronic cerebrospinal venous obstruction (CCSVO) refers to cerebrospinal venous blood flow disturbances with venous obstructions in the major extracranial veins of the head, neck, and vertebral column that predominantly affect the CSVS but may also involve the IJVs. The predominant pathology is chronic and constant obstruction of the major veins of the neck and vertebral column with resultant development of collateral flow and new pathways. The veins involved include the IJVs, VVs, external and internal vertebral venous plexuses, and azygous veins. CCSVO may be associated with a wide range of chronic vascular and inflammatory diseases, generally with manifestations in the head, neck, and chest [15, 16]. These include multiple sclerosis, rosacea, disfiguring dilated superficial veins in the head, neck, and chest, cervical spondylosis as well as chronic cough, chronic sinusitis, and chronic fatigue syndrome. The vague neurological symptoms of brain fog, poor cognition, headaches, and fatigue are common presenting symptoms of the syndrome.

The venous obstructions reduce the flow in the neck veins and can result in complete occlusion of these veins, most commonly affecting the vertebral veins and internal and external vertebral venous plexuses. Thibault [17] has suggested that these venous obstructions are due to a chronic persistent venulitis caused by the obligate, intracellular parasite, *Chlamydophila pneumoniae (Cpn)*. This parasitic bacterium has also been associated with other vascular diseases including coronary artery disease, cerebrovascular disease, late-onset vascular dementia, and aortic aneurysms [18].

In contrast, localized venous obstructions in the neck caused by apparent extrinsic compression, particularly affecting the IJVs, have also been reported [19]. IJV extrinsic compression at the passage between the C1 transverse process and the styloid process, presents with anatomical features of Eagle syndrome (an elongated styloid process impinging the surrounding blood vessels) and has been associated with intracranial hypertension and venous outflow reduction. The most frequent symptoms are headache, tinnitus, insomnia, visual disturbances, and localized pain is characteristic [20].

4. Extracranial duplex ultrasound examination of the neck veins

To accurately assess obstruction in the CSVS, Thibault and Lewis have developed a quantitative extracranial duplex ultrasound examination (ECDU) of the neck veins [14]. The method of the ECDU has been described in detail [14, 16]. To take advantage of the normal postural dependency of the venous outflow from the brain, venous obstruction is determined by comparing the venous blood volume flow (VBVF) measurements for the different segments of the vein examined (**Figure 2**) in the supine and erect positions. The sensitivity and specificity of the ECDU examination for the identification of stenoses in the IJVs have been calculated as 85% and 100%, respectively, by using venography as the gold standard [14].

Color-flow duplex ultrasound scanning is performed using a 7.5 MHz linear array multi-frequency transducer. The patients are examined supine (0°) with the head in a neutral position. Each IJV is visualized in a sagittal plane, lateral to the common carotid artery. The IJV is followed to its confluence with the subclavian and brachiocephalic veins at the base of the neck. In B-mode, the proximal IJV is assessed with anatomic

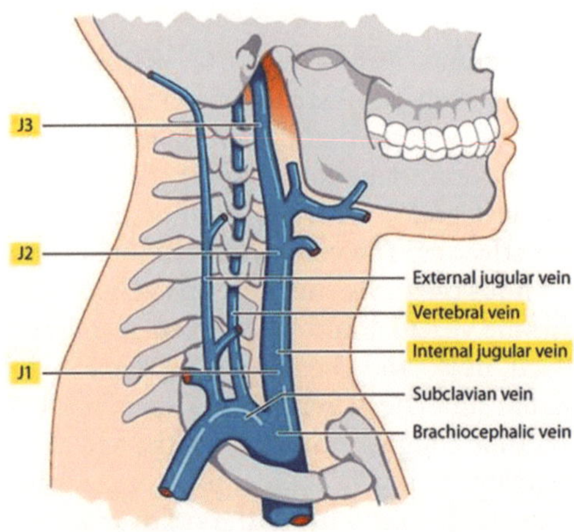

Figure 2.
Schematic diagram demonstrating venous blood volume flow (VBVF) measurement sites. J1: proximal internal jugular vein; J2 mid internal jugular vein; J3: distal internal jugular vein [14].

abnormalities, such as duplication and valvular malformations. Vein wall thickening can indicate present or past inflammation, and collaterals are recorded and mapped. Color Doppler is employed to demonstrate flow in the vein, the direction of flow, and turbulence. Stagnation of flow, defined as stationary blood that elicits no Doppler signal, is noted. Cephalad flow (reflux) is assessed during normal respiration. If the reversed flow is present on the pulsed or color Doppler signals, the time duration of reflux is measured on the pulsed Doppler tracing. Reflux is present if the duration exceeds 0.88 s [21]. Color Doppler assists in locating stenoses. Throughout the ECDU, the ultrasound transducer is lightly placed on the skin surface to avoid compression of the veins.

BVF measurements are obtained bilaterally from the proximal (J1), mid (J2), and distal (J3) IJV segments [22], and the mid-VVs (**Figure 2**). The J1 segment reading is generally discarded as it has demonstrated high variability in the BVF measurement at that level related to excessive turbulence close to the proximal valve [23]. If no or low flow is recorded in the VV, then another reading is taken distally as the segmental obstruction is frequently observed in the VVs. To record a BVF, the pulsed Doppler sample volume is placed in the center of the longitudinally imaged vein with a sample gate size the diameter of the vessel. Pulsed Doppler recordings are obtained over 3–5 cardiac cycles. With the Doppler spectrum frozen, the venous Doppler signal (**Figure 3**) is traced for 3–5 cardiac cycles. The cross-sectional area (CSA) is obtained by measuring the diameter of the vein at the location of the sample volume (**Figure 3**). The BVF is displayed and recorded in milliliters per minute (**Figure 3**).

When the examination is completed in the supine position, the patient is positioned in the seated position (90°) with the head in a neutral position looking directly ahead. The patient takes several deep inspirations and expirations and rests quietly for a 2-min period to allow for adaptation to the postural change before the commencement of the erect examination [24]. The right and left IJV and VVs are re-assessed for valvular competence, reflux, stenosis or thrombosis, external compression, and stagnation of flow. BVF measurements of the J1, J2, and J3 segments of the IJV and mid-cervical VVs

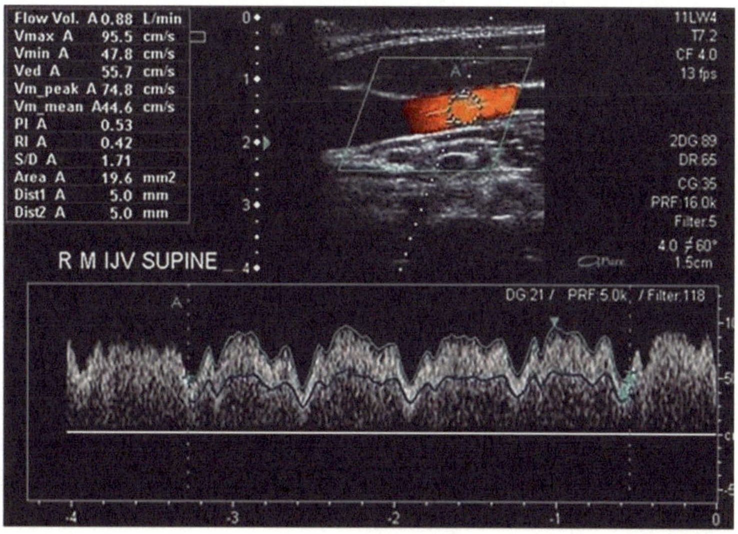

Figure 3.
Duplex ultrasound image with color doppler demonstrating measurement of BVF in the J2 segment of an IJV by calculating the circular CSA of the vein with BVF averaged over 3–5 cardiac cycles in the supine position. The BVF measurement obtained from the J2 segment IJV shows an abnormally high-flow rate of 880 ml/min [14].

Supine	Flow volumes right (ml/min)	Flow volumes left (ml/min)
IJV (J1)	836	346
IJV (J2)	400	154
IJV (J3)	266	37
Vertebral	7	17
Int. Carotid A.	279	482
Vertebral A.	53	60
Global Arterial Cerebral Blood Flow 874 mls/min		
Sitting		
IJV (J1)	1317	46
IJV (J2)	249	41
IJV (J3)	349	0
Vertebral	82	61

Table 1.
Typical worksheet detailing the BVF measurements obtained in the extracranial duplex ultrasound (ECDU) examination [14]. This worksheet indicates distal L IJV obstruction, with collateral flow through the R IJV (erect) possibly indicating some CSVO.

are repeated. The measurements for the erect position are taken at the same positions as the supine measurements. A typical BVF worksheet is shown in **Table 1**.

The loss of normal postural change in the VBVF reading is suggestive of obstruction in either the jugular venous system or the CSVS. Note that detection of obstruction in the CSVS depends on direct measurement of VV BF (in either or both positions) and corresponding increased IJV BF in the erect position where normally the IJV collapses with a corresponding 10-fold reduction in BF compared with the supine position [12]. If there is CSVO, there will usually be increased collateral flow through the IJV on the same side and occasionally through the VV of the opposite side. If there is unilateral obstruction of an IJV, there will be increased flow through the IJV of the opposite side, increased flow through the VV of the same side, or the presence of collaterals including increased flow in the external jugular vein. Obstruction in the vertebral venous plexuses cannot be measured directly by ultrasonography, however, can be inferred if the IJV flows are increased in the erect position when the VV BFs are normal.

Chambers et al. in their study [25], suggested that normal results may be defined according to 10th and 90th percentiles (**Table 2**).

It is possible for the L IJV to be compressed completely in the erect position with no other abnormality observed. However, Zamboni [22] has stated that no flow in any segment in any position is abnormal. Therefore, in the situation of an isolated IJV segment showing no flow in the erect position, the probability of abnormality should be based on the presence of abnormal collateral flow (**Table 1**, L IJV erect position with collateral flow through R IJV). Abnormal patterns of flow manifested by the VBVFs should be consistent over time in the same patient but may show signs of improvement with treatment or deterioration with the progression of the disorder.

Clinical practice guidelines have been developed to interpret the VBVFs in the ECDU of neck veins based on previously published data of "normal" subjects [10–13], and the author's clinical experience in assessing abnormalities in neck vein venous flow using

	Supine		Sitting	
	Patients	**Controls**	**Patients**	**Controls**
Right				
J1[a]	531 (219, 980)	634 (241, 848)	891 (238, 1403)	457 (162, 937)
J2	354 (181, 477)	371 (221, 614)	203 (94, 382)	177 (64, 418)
J3	259 (129, 429)	393 (215, 622)	161 (55, 259)	131 (68, 272)
VV	44 (21, 63)	35 (19, 59)	103 (51, 180)	101 (44, 226)
Left				
J1[a]	332 (57, 640)	356 (164, 618)	324 (98, 635)	345 (109, 1143)
J2	258 (174, 476)	261 (144, 431)	119 (61, 330)	134 (72, 357)
J3	171 (109, 332)	179 (110, 297)	73 (25, 155)	72 (29, 192)
VV	28 (18, 47)	27 (15, 46)	87 (51, 72)	76 (50, 131)

J1: inferior internal jugular vein; J2: mid internal jugular vein; J3: superior internal jugular vein; VV: vertebral vein.[a]J1 values excluded in the first 24 cases.

Table 2.
Median (and interquartile range) volume flow values (mL/s) in early MS patients and controls [13].

	High (mL/min)	Normal (mL/min)	Low (mL/min)
Right supine			
IJV J2	>750	150–750	<150
IJV J3	>600	100–600	<100
VV	>90	20–90	<20
Sitting			
IJV J2	>170	30–170	<30
IJV J3	>150	10–150	<10
VV	>250	70–250	<70
Left supine			
IJV J2	>600	100–600	<100
IJV J3	>400	80–400	<80
VV	>70	20–70	<20
Sitting			
IJV J2	>170	20–170	<20
IJV J3	>150	10–150	<10
VV	>250	70–250	<70

Table 3.
BVF guidelines to diagnosing abnormalities in neck vein blood flow [16].

this examination (**Table 3**). If there is borderline flow in the VVs in the erect position, the probability of abnormality is increased if there is increased collateral flow in the ipsilateral IJV in the erect position signifying obstruction somewhere in the CSVS.

5. CCSVO and chronic infective venulitis

A chronic infective venulitis involving persistent *Cpn* infection was first published in 2012 [17]. The spread of *Cpn* from the lungs to the vasculature has been demonstrated by Geiffers et al. [26] *Cpn* infection of the lungs results in interstitial and alveolar pneumonia with bronchiolitis that resolves spontaneously after 2–4 weeks.

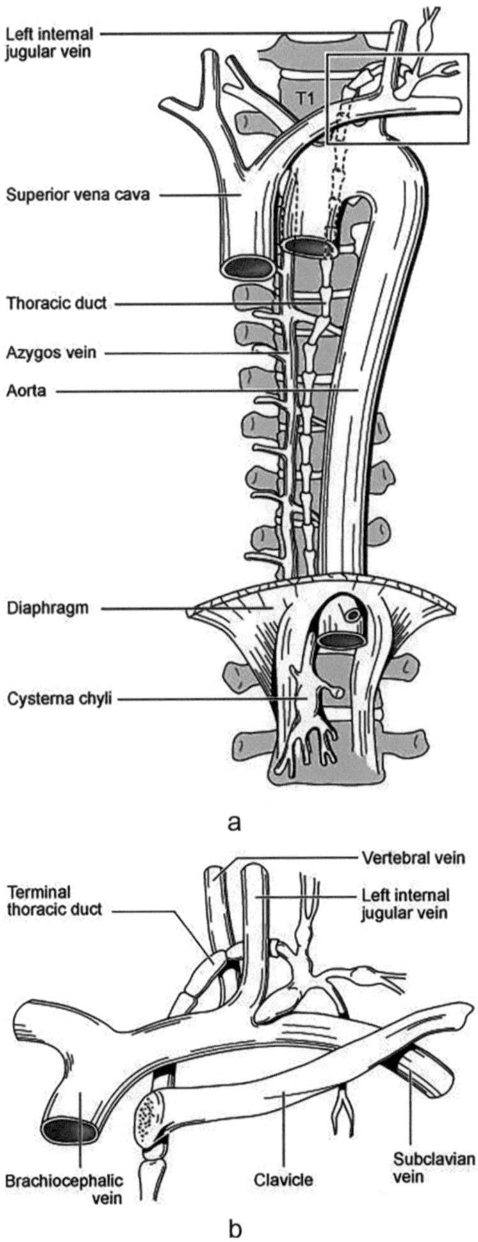

Figure 4.
(a) Relative anatomy of the thoracic duct. Note the close association of the thoracic duct to the azygos vein on the thoracic spine. (b) the termination of the thoracic duct at the confluence of the subclavian vein, left internal jugular vein, and left vertebral vein. Infected macrophages and lymphocytes with C. pneumoniae transmit the infection to the venous endothelium at this site, triggering a creeping venulitis to affect the cerebrospinal venous system (CSVS) [17].

Histology reveals infiltrates of heterophilic granulocytes and mononuclear cells within the lungs. There is often mild vasculitis and perivasculitis within the first 3 days. Perivascular and peribronchiolar lymphatic hyperplasia is observed from day three until up to 8 weeks from the initial infection. The monocytes are unable to eliminate the *Cpn* organism and carry the *Cpn* through the lymphatic system. *Cpn* organisms are thereby transmitted through peri-hilar lymph nodes to the thoracic duct and right lymphatic duct. From these lymphatic pathways, the monocytes transmit the *Cpn* elementary bodies (EBs) to the venous endothelium, firstly, through communications of the thoracic duct with the azygos vein in the chest, then at the confluences of the internal jugular, vertebral, and subclavian veins bilaterally (**Figure 4a** and **b**). Once blood-borne, the *Cpn* can also spread to distant vascular sites carried by the infected blood monocytes [27]. Aided by the presence of platelets, *Cpn*-infected monocytes exhibit increased adhesion to vascular endothelial cells [28] and *Cpn* activation of chemokines in human endothelial cells promotes peri-vascular inflammation [29].

The infective venulitis theory was originally developed to explain the neck vein abnormalities found in subjects with MS [17]. *Cpn* rapidly binds to platelets causing platelet activation, aggregation, ATP secretion, and surface expression of P-selectin [30]. P-selectin mediates the recruitment and activation of leukocytes and thereby initiates an inflammatory response [30]. *Cpn* is transferred to the endothelial linings of these vessels when *Cpn*-infected monocytes come into contact with platelets in the venous blood of the cerebrospinal venous system. A creeping infective venulitis then spreads slowly and silently within the cerebrospinal venous system, including the IJVs. The lymphatic ducts remain unaffected owing to the absence of platelets in the lymph. Over time, the prothrombotic and inflammatory effects of the *Cpn* venulitis cause gradual obstruction of the VVs and vertebral venous plexuses, although the IJVs can also become affected despite their larger diameter. Pathology studies of abnormal valves in IJVs in patients with MS have shown an absence of endothelial cells where a reticular and fibrotic lamina has replaced the endothelium suggesting a past, resolved inflammatory or thrombotic process that involved the wall of the IJV [31].

From the chest and neck, *Cpn* can be transmitted to other blood vessels throughout the body via infected monocytes to cause arterial and venous inflammation that could play a significant role in chronic vascular diseases. PCR testing of atheromatous vessels in the chest (aorta, coronary arteries, and internal mammary arteries) and macroscopically abnormal great saphenous veins have been found to be positive for *Cpn*, whereas normal vessels in the same subjects have been negative indicating that *Cpn* has a role in both atheromatous changes in arteries and degenerative changes in veins [32, 33]. Studies confirm the presence of *Cpn* in atheromatous coronary arteries and other major arteries. Also, serological studies confirm that the presence of *Cpn* antibodies increases the risk of vascular disease [34]. The mechanisms by which *Cpn* promotes vascular diseases and stimulates immune and inflammatory responses are well understood, and it is, therefore, likely that persistent *Cpn* is a risk factor in cardiovascular disease and venous diseases characterized by chronic inflammation [35].

6. Laboratory evidence of chronic persistent *Cpn* infection

6.1 Serology

Chlamydophila pneumoniae was first isolated by Grayston et al. [36] in 1965 and was identified as a separate species of the genus Chlamydia in 1989. This primary respiratory obligate intracellular parasite has the capacity to infect and multiply within a wide range of secondary host cells, including macrophages, lymphocytes, and vascular endothelial cells [36]. The primary infection with *Cpn* does not induce life-long immunity with most individuals having several infections during their lifetime. Subsequent re-infections with *Cpn* induce a greater IgG response than the initial infection. Small children do not frequently produce IgA antibodies as a response to primary upper respiratory tract infections with *Cpn,* but IgA responses are generally more common in re-infections, which are more common in adults [37, 38]. By the age of 20 years, 50% of people have antibodies to *Cpn*. The prevalence of antibodies increases with age, reaching a peak in seropositivity of 80% in men and 70% in women by age 65 [39, 40]. Grayston [41] suggested that eventually everyone becomes infected with *Cpn.*

Because of the high prevalence of antibodies present in adults, the relevance of persistent *Cpn* infection serological testing alone does not reliably indicate the presence of clinically significant persistent *Cpn*. Persistently elevated IgG or the presence of IgA antibodies have been frequently used to identify persons with persistent or chronic infections [42]. High IgA titers may be a better marker of chronic *Cpn* infection than IgG titers because serum IgA has a half-life of 5–7 days, whereas IgG has a half-life of weeks to months. Therefore, ideally, a healthy person free from *Cpn* venulitis should not exhibit IgA antibodies. However, the use of serological testing as a stand-alone test to define patients as "persistently infected" must await further validation [43].

6.2 Dyslipidemia

Cpn antibodies have been associated with an atherogenic lipid profile in men [44]. Finnish men who tested positive for *Cpn* IgG had significantly higher triglyceride concentrations and lower HDL than seronegative subjects [45].

In laboratory mice, *Cpn* liver infection induces dyslipidemia by modifying genes involved in lipid metabolism [46]. *Cpn*-infected mice show significantly increased cholesterol and triglyceride levels compared with negative controls and *Chlamydia trachomatis* infected mice. In *Cpn*-infected livers, cholesterol 7α-hydroxylase and low-density lipoprotein receptor (LDLr) mRNA levels are reduced, while inducible degrader of the LDLr expression is increased.

Cpn-infected macrophages ingest excess LDL to become cholesterol-laden foam cells, creating early lesions in athero-sclerosis [47]. In addition, *Cpn* induces monocytes to oxidize lipoproteins, converting them to highly atherogenic forms [48]. As well as causing increased platelet aggregation, *Cpn* interaction with platelets results in reactive oxygen species (ROS) causing oxidative damage on LDL [49]. *Cpn*-induced foam cell formation is mediated chiefly by lipopolysaccharide, whereas lipoprotein oxidation occurs mainly by chlamydial heat shock protein 60 (cHSP60), an inflammatory protein expressed by persistent chlamydiae [34]. In addition cHSP60 may contribute to atherogenesis by triggering antibody-mediated cytotoxicity through an immunological cross-reactivity to HSP60 produced by the infected endothelial cell [50]. One of the similar mechanisms whereby *Cpn* can trigger demyelination lesions found in MS is by direct toxic effects of HSP60 and activation of innate immunity [51–53].

6.3 C-reactive protein (CRP) as an inflammatory marker

CRP is an acute-phase protein that serves as an early marker of inflammation or infection. During bacterial infection or inflammatory disease states, CRP levels rise rapidly within the first 6–8 hours and peak at levels of up to 350–400 mg/L after 48 h. Highly sensitive (hs)CRP is an independent risk factor for cardiovascular disease. The risk of developing cardiovascular disease is quantified as follows [54]:

- low: CRP level under 1.0 mg/L
- average: between 1.0 and 3.0 mg/L
- high: above 3.0 mg/L.

There is a correlation between the elevation of serum CRP and the presence of *Cpn* in carotid and coronary artery atheromatous plaques [55–58]. There is also a strong correlation between serum *Cpn* IgA and serum CRP levels in subjects with known vascular disease [57, 58]. Specific antibiotic treatment for chronic persistent *Cpn* infection in subjects with the vascular disease has resulted in a significant reduction in CRP levels at 6-month follow-up [59]. When the inflammation or tissue destruction is resolved, CRP levels fall, making it a useful marker for monitoring disease activity [60]. When monitoring the effectiveness of treatment of persistent *Cpn* infection, hsCRP levels of less than 1.0 mg/L are aimed for.

6.4 Liver dysfunction

Cpn is known to infect the liver, generally in association with the presence of cardiovascular disease [61]. In addition *Cpn* has been implicated in primary biliary cirrhosis [62] and granulomatous hepatitis [63]. It is known that *Cpn* acute liver infection affects cholesterol and triglyceride metabolism, as described previously [46]. *Cpn* has been demonstrated to survive and replicate in Kupffer cells of the liver thereby creating a chronic hepatitis [64].

Cpn can infect the liver, and therefore liver function tests can be abnormal. ALT has been associated with a greater probability of a positive serology result for *Cpn*, therefore, may be a useful diagnostic marker for the disease [65]. In addition both AST and GGT can be elevated in patients with chronic *Cpn* infection.

6.5 Abnormal serum iron (Fe) studies

Many bacteria, including *Cpn*, are dependent on iron (Fe) for their growth. One of the first lines of immune defense against bacterial infection is the withholding of Fe to prevent bacterial multiplication [66]. Fe restriction in cell culture inhibits the growth of *Cpn* [67]. Circulating hormone hepcidin, produced by the liver, acts as a regulator of body Fe homeostasis. During infection and inflammation, hepcidin production is induced, driving a decrease in Fe concentration by inhibiting the absorption of Fe and promoting the sequestration of Fe in macrophages and the liver [68].

Liver hepcidin levels in mice increase during acute *Cpn* infection and this induction is associated with altered Fe levels [69]. Serum Fe levels decrease during the course of a *Cpn infection* in mice [70]. In a chronic persistent *Cpn* infection, low-to-normal serum Fe levels associated with mild to moderately elevated serum ferritin levels are frequently observed. If found to be elevated initially, serum ferritin levels can be a useful parameter to measure response to treatment of chronic persistent *Cpn* infection. Similarly low serum Fe levels at the onset of treatment should respond by increasing to normal levels during the course of treatment. Low transferrin levels are also a nonspecific indicator of chronic systemic infection and can be used to monitor the success of treatment.

7. Requirements for diagnosis of chronic persistent *Cpn*

There have been many epidemiological, microbiological, serological, and histological studies that suggest that *Cpn* may play a role in the pathogenesis of some chronic vascular and inflammatory diseases [71]. Chronic persistent *Cpn* infection creates pathological abnormalities that can be detected by targeted investigations. These include the ECDU examination in addition to the pathology tests outlined above. A normal ECDU will generally exclude a diagnosis of chronic persistent *Cpn* vasculitis. In most cases, the predictive power of a positive diagnosis will be attained if the triad of the presence of CCSVO as determined by the ECDU, positive serology (particularly if *Cpn* IgA is present), and dyslipidemia is attained. Secondary supporting evidence consists of elevation of serum CRP above 3.0 mg/L, elevated ALT and/or AST, and abnormal Fe studies.

Successful treatment of chronic persistent *Cpn* is recognized to be difficult and entails a multimodal therapy including a prolonged antibiotic protocol, usually for at least 6 months, dietary measures, specific supplements, and long-term control of dyslipidemia. Therefore, the certainty of diagnosis is essential.

8. Treatment of chronic persistent *Cpn* Venulitis

Cpn has a unique triphasic life cycle with a smaller extracellular form, which is the elementary body (EB), and a larger intracellular form, which is the reticulate body (RB) that can replicate. Under pressure from host defenses, the metabolic processes of the organism are diminished and in this nonreplicating state, called the cryptic or persistent form (CF), the organism can ensure intracellular persistence (**Figure 5**) [72, 73].

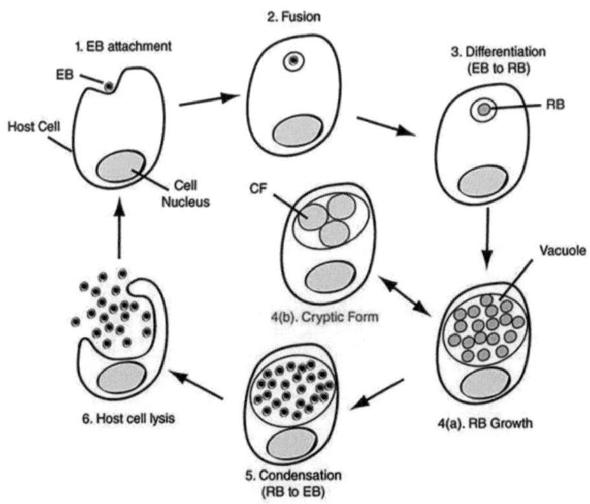

Figure 5.
The triphasic Chlamydophila pneumoniae lifecycle [15].

Because of this life cycle and various physiological mechanisms of the organism, short courses of single antibiotics have been shown to be ineffective in eliminating *Cpn* from infected tissues [75]. In addition, first-line antibiotic therapeutics induce persistence of *Cpn* [73]. Antibiotics that have been found to be effective against the RB include minocycline and doxycycline, and macrolides, such as clarithromycin and roxithromycin [76]. The EB may be sensitive to N-acetyl-cysteine (NAC) and the CF is sensitive to tinidazole and metronidazole [76, 77]. Due to the inherent ability of the chlamydial organism to persist in infected tissues [78], a combined antibiotic protocol (CAP) has been described that addresses all three forms of the chlamydial lifecycle to minimize persistence of the organism [77]. The strategy of this protocol is to induce the persistent form from the RB by using a combination of tetracycline and a macrolide and then kill the CF with intermittent pulses of tinidazole or metronidazole [74]. In addition, disruption of the outer membrane proteins of EBs by constant exposure to NAC initiates the transition of the EB form to the RB form, which is susceptible to the tetracycline/macrolide combination [77].

The effect of a CAP directed at treating the persistent infection with *Cpn* on the manifestation of CCSVO observed in MS as measured by ECDU has been investigated [15]. A non-randomized before-after cohort study was conducted to investigate differences in VBVF pre- and post-CAP treatment of *Cpn* infection.

Ninety-one consecutive patients presenting with MS were investigated for the presence of circulating *Cpn* antibodies and CCSVO. There were 64 females and 27 males, aged from 20 to 71 included in the study. Thirty-six had been classified as relapsing–remitting (RR) MS, 39 as secondary progressive (SP), and 16 were primary progressive (PP).

ECDU was performed as previously described [14]. *Cpn* status was defined as having a positive reading on either *Cpn* IgG or *Cpn* IgA using an automated ELIZA analyzer. The vascular sonographer was blinded as to each individual subject's *Cpn* serology status.

Blood volume flow (BVF) data from the 91 patients were measured across affected and unaffected sides from multiple vein segments (J2, J3, and VV) (**Figure 2**). Owing to the known postural changes that occur in the IJVs and VVs[10–12] J2 and J3 readings were recorded in the supine position, whereas VV readings were recorded in the erect position. A side (right or left) was considered affected if one or more of the BVFs from J2, J3, or VV were below the reference range described in **Table 3**. Overall, 40 subjects had bilateral "affected" sides, 45 had unilateral "affected" sides, and six had neither side "affected."

All patients were treated with a CAP for 6 months then had repeat ECDU to assess response. The sonographer was blinded as to the "affected" or "unaffected" status of each vein segment at the 6-month follow-up examination.

The CAP consisted of minocycline 50–100 mg twice daily according to patient weight, roxithromycin 150 mg twice daily, tinidazole 500 mg twice daily for 2 days each month, and NAC 1200 mg twice daily. This protocol is based on that advised by Stratton and Wheldon [72, 75].

The advantage of this study was that it incorporated two within-subject controls (un-affected side and pre-post comparisons) and a between-subjects control (no *Cpn* antibodies). A test of differences was performed pooling results across all vein segments (J2, J3, and VV). The parameters of the linear mixed model were estimated, and the least-squares means are shown in **Figure 6**.

There was a statistically significant posttreatment difference seen for the affected side of *Cpn* positive serology patients (mean difference = 56 mls/min, $p = 0.02$, 95%

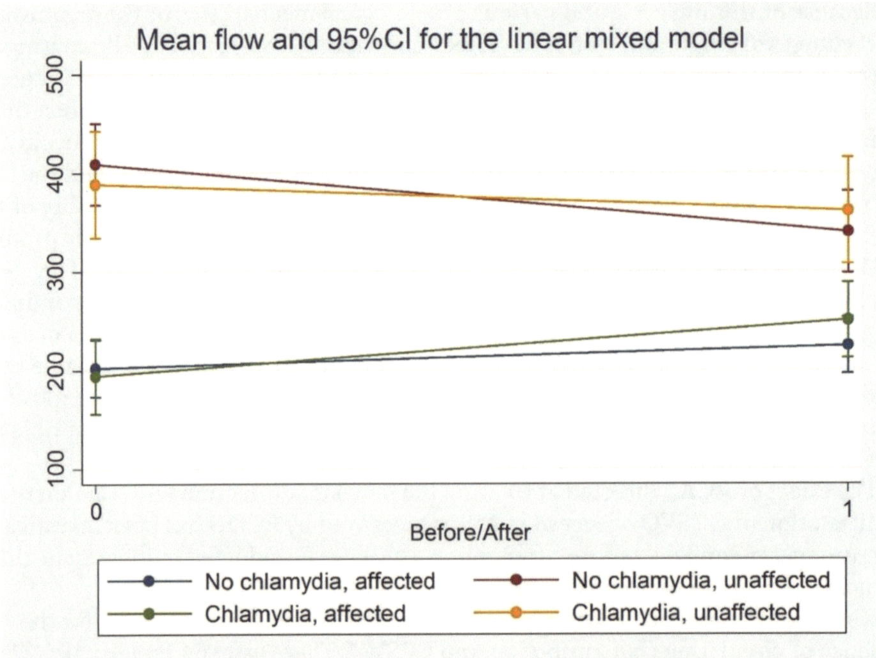

Figure 6.
Mean values pooled over three vein segments over time [15].

CI: 8, 105). There was a smaller increase seen for the affected side of negative serology patients (mean difference = 23 mls/min, 95%C I: −13, 59) and not statistically significant (p = 0.2). The difference in these effects (34 mls/min, 95% CI: −27, 94) was not statistically significant (p = 0.3). The mean flow rate decreased in the unaffected side for both positive serology patients (−27 mls/min, p = 0.5, 95% CI: −98, 44 mls/min) and negative serology patients (−69 mls/min, p = 0.012, 95% CI: −123, −115 mls/min).

This study demonstrated that obstructed VBF in the major extracranial veins of the neck in subjects with MS can be improved by a prolonged CAP, specifically designed to treat persistent *Cpn* infection. This effect was significant in those subjects that tested positive with *Cpn* serology. The improved blood flow in the affected veins was consistently associated with a corresponding reduction in collateral flow in the unaffected side in those subjects with unilateral disease. Although there was no significant difference between positive and negative serology patients, this is consistent with the known sensitivity of around 70% for the *Cpn* serology tests [79].

9. Supplementary and ongoing treatments for CCSVO

The ability of *Cpn* to persist despite antimicrobial therapy with agents to which it is susceptible *in vitro* is well documented [76]. Therefore other strategies are required for long-term control of persistent *Cpn* infection:

1. **Statins (coenzyme A reductase inhibitors).** *Cpn* does not have the capacity to synthesize cholesterol, but cholesterol is required for its intracellular multiplication

and is an essential component of the chlamydial spore [80]. Thus *Cpn* is dependent on the availability of host cholesterol inside the cell where it replicates. *Cpn* may use cholesterol derived either from the extracellular space via low-density lipoprotein uptake or from intracellular cholesterol stores. By reducing cholesterol levels, statins may affect chlamydial intracell multiplication [81]. Erkkilä and colleagues [80] were also able to demonstrate that simvastatin amplified pulmonary inflammatory response by increasing inflammatory cell infiltration into the lungs during acute *Cpn* infection in mice. Therefore, statin treatment may have an anti-*Cpn* effect *in vivo*.

2. **Berberine.** Berberine is an isoquinoline alkaloid isolated from the bark, roots, rhizome, and stems of plants of the genus *Berberis*, as well as from plants, such as *Coptis chinensis* and *Hydrastis canadensis* (goldenseal). Berberine has been found to lower lipid levels by a different mechanism than that of statins. It is thought to upregulate the expression of LDL receptors (LDLR) on hepatocytes by stabilizing LDLR mRNA [82]. Preliminary animal and pilot human studies have shown that berberine produces a positive effect on the lipid profile both on its own and as an adjunct to simvastatin [83, 84].

In addition, one of the mechanisms that *Cpn* contributes to the development of atherosclerosis is by promoting vascular smooth muscle cell (VSMC) migration. It has been shown that berberine inhibits *Cpn* infection-induced VSMC migration by downregulating the expressions of the matrix metalloproteinases MMP3 and MMP9 [85].

3. **Resveratrol.** It has been shown that *Cpn* is able to promote the accumulation of low-density lipoproteins into macrophages, thus facilitating foam cell formation. Resveratrol is a plant polyphenol commonly found in red wine. Di Pietro and colleagues [86] were able to show an antiatherogenic effect of resveratrol on macrophage-derived foam cell formation induced by *Cpn*. Resveratrol has also been shown to inhibit reactive oxygen species production by directly decreasing NADP oxidase (NOX) activity [86, 87]. Furthermore resveratrol has been shown to inhibit the growth of *Cpn* in presence of clarithromycin or ofloxacin compared to controls [88]. This suggested that the combined treatment of an appropriate antibiotic with resveratrol may afford a synergistic effect in controlling *Cpn* infections.

4. **Disulfiram.** For patients that fail to respond to the recommended therapeutic suggestions (see Appendix), the use of Disulfiram should be considered. Disulfiram is used as a deterrent to promote abstinence in chronic alcoholism treatment. In the body, Disulfiram and its metabolites inhibit aldehyde dehydrogenase (ALDH) by thiol-disulfide exchange with cysteine residues [89]. Irreversible inhibition of hepatic ALDH results in the bodily accumulation of toxic acetaldehyde produced during ethanol metabolism and an amplified "hangover" effect after alcohol is consumed [90].

Disulfiram also forms disulfides with thiol-bearing substances that can modify bacterial thiol-disulfide exchange to evoke antimicrobial effects [91]. For this reason it has been recently reported as being effective in treating multi-resistant staphylococcus infections [91] and chronic Borreliosis [92].

For the treatment of chronic *Cpn* infection, disulfiram can be used at a dose of 4 mg/kg/day combined with either minocycline or a macrolide for a period of 2–3 months. It should not be used with either tinidazole or metronidazole. Treatment should be commenced at a starting daily dose of 100 mg per day and slowly titrated up to the full dose (300–400 mg per day) over a period of 3–4 weeks. If the patient develops any signs suggestive of peripheral neuropathy, then disulfiram should be ceased immediately as this will allow spontaneous resolution of those symptoms.

10. Resolution of symptoms and signs with treatment

Symptoms should begin to improve within 1 month of commencing treatment, but this is highly variable. Initially, vague neurological symptoms such as brain fog and poor cognition improve, followed by improvement in fatigue and general energy levels. Chronic cough, headaches, and rosacea also improve early. This should be accompanied by improvement in abnormal blood tests, such as liver function tests (ALT, AST), increase in serum Fe levels with a corresponding decrease in elevated serum ferritin (if abnormal initially), and a progressive reduction in inflammatory markers (CRP). Serum lipids should be checked at 3 months and if cholesterol and/or LDL levels remain elevated above the target levels (4.5 and 2.5 mmol/L, respectively), then a statin, such as either rosuvastatin or simvastatin, should be introduced at a low dose initially and then titrated every 3 months to achieve an LDL around 2 mmol/L. The addition of berberine appears to help attain this goal.

Cpn serology should be repeated every 3 months aiming for complete elimination of any level of IgA antibodies (if present initially), as this goal appears to be related to achieving successful symptomatic improvement. Finally, the ECDU should be repeated at 6 months and periodically thereafter if clinically indicated, to assess response with the CCSVO. If there is failure to respond, consider a change in the macrolide or introduction of a course of disulfiram.

Generally, the aim is to suspend the CAP at 6 months and continue long-term treatment with statin, berberine, and resveratrol. This timetable, however, needs to be adapted to individual patient responses and requirements. Flexibility in management is essential.

Appendix: Thibault Combined Antibiotic Protocol (CAP)

For Persistent *Chlamydophila pneumoniae* (*CPn*) Infection Associated with Chronic Diseases/CCSVO.

1. **Minocycline** 50–100 mg twice daily. The alternative to minocycline is doxycycline 50–100 mg twice daily. Lower doses may be advised for lower body weights.

2. **Tinidazole** 500–1000 mg as a stat dose once a week. The alternative is metronidazole 400–800 mg twice a day once a week. Commence 1 week after starting minocycline or doxycycline. Initially commence on the lower dose and titrate up to the higher dose if clinically indicated.

3. **Roxithromycin** 150 mg twice daily, or 300 mg once daily commencing 2 weeks after starting minocycline or doxycycline. An alternative macrolide

is clarithromycin 250 mg twice a day dose. The macrolide acts synergistically with the tetracycline.

4. **Berberine** 500 mg twice daily. Berberine has a beneficial effect on dyslipidemia.

5. **Resveratrol** 250 mg twice a day. Resveratrol augments the effectiveness of the antibiotics and has antioxidant effects.

6. **Statin.** Generally, this will be required, and it is suggested that the statin should be commenced at a low dose 3 months after starting the antibiotic therapy. Either simvastatin 20–40 mg daily or in more resistant cases of dyslipidemia, rosuvastatin 5–40 mg daily is recommended. Fasting serum LDL cholesterol should be kept below 2.5 mmol. Lowering cholesterol starves the *Cpn* of cholesterol, a substance it acquires from the host cell to make the bacterial cell wall.

7. **Quercetin** 500 mg twice a day. This is recommended but not essential. Quercetin may augment the effect of the macrolide with *Cpn* and it has anti-inflammatory and antioxidant effects that may be beneficial to vascular endothelium.

8. **Diet** Complex carbohydrate, low-fat diet (paleolithic) avoiding milk and red meats. Avoid excessive alcohol.

9. **Vitamin D** 1000 IU twice daily. Serum vitamin D levels are frequently low in these patients. Deficiency in vitamin D is associated with increased susceptibility to infection.

10. **Vitamin B12 supplements.** These can be beneficial in patients with chronic fatigue

The initial treatment is generally for 6 months. After that, treatment may be reduced to a maintenance program (statin, resveratrol, and berberine) if deemed to be appropriate to prevent relapse.

Author details

Paul K. Thibault
Australasian College of Phlebology, Sydney, Australia

*Address all correspondence to: paul@cvcmc.net

References

[1] Tobinick E, Vega CP. The cerebrospinal venous system: Anatomy, physiology, and clinical implications. MedGenMed. 2006;**8**(1):53

[2] Batson OV. The function of the vertebral veins and their role in the spread of metastases. Annals of Surgery. 1940;**112**:138-149

[3] Breschet G. Recherches Anatomiques Physiologiques et Pathologiques Sur le systáeme Veineux. Rouen fráeres: Paris, France; 1829

[4] Groen RJ, du Toit DF, Phillips FM, et al. Anatomical and pathological considerations in percutaneous vertebroplasty and kyphoplasty: A reappraisal of the vertebral venous system. Spine. 2004;**29**:1465-1471

[5] Groen RJ, Groenewegen HJ, van Alphen HA, et al. Morphology of the internal vertebral venous plexus; a cadaver study after intravenous araldite CY 221 injection. The Anatomical Record. 1997;**86**:252-262

[6] Chou CH, Chao AC, Hu HH. Ultrasonographic of vertebral venous valves. AJNR. American Journal of Neuroradiology. 2002;**23**:1418-1420

[7] Osborn AGO. Craniofacial venous plexuses.: Angiographic study. AJR. American Journal of Roentgenology. 1981;**136**:139-143

[8] Batson OV. The vertebral vein system. Caldwell lecture, 1956. The American Journal of Roentgenology, Radium Therapy, and Nuclear Medicine. 1957;**78**:195-212

[9] Epstein HM, Linde HW, Crompton AR, Cine IS, Eckenholf JJE. The vertebral venous plexus as a major cerebral venous outflow tract. Anesthesiology. 1970;**32**:332-340. DOI: 10.1097/00000542-197004000-00007

[10] Doepp F, Schreiber SJ, von Münster T, Rademacher J, Klingebiel R, Valdueza JM. How does the blood leave the brain? A systematic ultrasound analysis of cerebral venous drainage patterns. Neuroradiology. 2004;**46**:565-570

[11] Schreiber SJ, Lürtzing F, Gotze R, Doepp F, et al. Extrajugular pathways of human cerebral venous blood drainage assessed by duplex ultrasound. Journal of Applied Physiology. 2003;**4**:1802-1805

[12] Valdueza JM, von Münster T, Hoffmann O, Schreiber S, Einhäupl KM. Postural dependency of the cerebral venous outflow. Lancet. 2000;**355**:200-201

[13] Chambers B, Chambers J, Churilov L. Internal jugular and vertebral vein volume flow in patients with clinically isolated syndrome or mild multiple sclerosis and healthy controls: Results from a prospective sonographer-blinded study. Phlebology. 2014;**29**:528-535

[14] Thibault P, Lewis W, Niblett S. Objective duplex ultrasound examination of the extracranial circulation in patients undergoing venoplasty of internal jugular vein stenosis: A pilot study. Phlebology. 2015;**30**:98-104

[15] Thibault P, Attia J, Oldmeadow C. A prolonged antibiotic protocol to treat persistent *Chlamydophila pneumoniae* infection improves the extracranial venous circulation in multiple sclerosis. Phlebology. 2018;**33**(6):397-406

[16] Thibault PK. Neck vein obstruction: Diagnosis and the role of chronic

persistent Chlamydophila pneumoniae infection. Phlebology. 2019;**34**(6):372-379. DOI: 10.1177/0268355518804379

[17] Thibault PK. Multiple sclerosis: A chronic infective cerebrospinal venulitis? Phlebology. 2012;**27**:207-218

[18] Ouellette SP, Byrne GI. *Chlamydia pneumoniae*: Prospects and predictions for an emerging pathogen. In: *Chlamydia pneumoniae*: Infection and Disease. 2004. DOI: 10.1007/0-306-48741-1. ISBN: 978-0-306-48487-2

[19] Scerrati A, Norri N, Mongardi L, Dones F, Ricciardi L, Trevisi G, et al. Styloidogenic-cervical spondylotic internal jugular venous compression, a vascular disease related to several clinical neurological manifestations: diagnosis and treatment-a comprehensive literature review. The Annals of Translational Medicine's. 2021 Apr;**9**(8):718. DOI: 10.21037/atm-20-7698

[20] Zamboni P, Scerrati A, Menegatti E et al. The eagle jugular syndrome. BMC Neurology. 2019;**19**:333. DOI: 10.1186/s12883-019-1572-3

[21] Menagatti E, Zamboni P. Doppler haemodynamics of cerebral venous return. Current Neurovascular Research. 2008;**5**:260-265

[22] Zamboni P, Morovic S, Menegatti E. Screening for chronic cerebrospinal venous insufficiency (CCSVI) using ultrasound: Recommendations for a protocol. International Angiology. 2011;**30**:571-597

[23] Zamboni P. Why current Doppler ultrasound methodology is inaccurate in assessing cerebral venous return: The alternative of the ultrasonic jugular venous pulse. Behavioural Neurology 2016;**2016**:7082856. DOI: 10.1155/2016/7082856

[24] Zamboni P, Galeotti R, Menegatti E. Chronic cerebrospinal venous insufficiency in patients with multiple sclerosis. Journal of Neurology, Neurosurgery, and Psychiatry. 2009;**80**:392-399

[25] Chambers B, Chambers J, Churilov L. Internal jugular and vertebral vein volume flow in patients with clinically isolated syndrome or mild multiple sclerosis and healthy controls: Results from a prospective sonographer-blinded study. Phlebology. 2014;**29**:528-535

[26] Geiffers J, van Zandbergan G, Rupp J. Phagocytes transmit Chlamydophila pneumonia from the lungs to the vasculature. The European Respiratory Journal. 2004;**23**:506-510

[27] Cole WR, Witte MH, Witte CL. Lymph culture: A new tool for the investigation of human infections. Annals of Surgery. 1969;**170**:705-713

[28] Kalayoglu MV, Perkins BN, Byrne GI. *Chlamydia pneumoniae*-infected monocytes exhibit increased adherence to human aortic endothelial cells. Microbes and Infection. 2001;**3**:963-969

[29] Molestina RE, Miller RD, Ramirez JA. Infection of human endothelial cells with *chlamydia pneumoniae* stimulates transendothelial migration of neutrophils and monoctyes. Infection and Immunity. 1999;**67**:1323-1330

[30] Kälvegren H, Majeed M, Bengtsson T. *Chlamydia pneumoniae* binds to platelets and triggers P-selectin expression and aggregation: A causal role in cardiovascular disease? Arteriosclerosis, Thrombosis, and Vascular Biology. 2003;**23**:1677-1683

[31] Zamboni P, Tisato V, Menegatti E. Ultrastructure of internal jugular

vein defective valves. Phlebology. 2015;**30**:644-647

[32] Taylor-Robinson D, Thomas BJ. *Chlamydia pneumoniae* in atherosclerotic tissue. The Journal of Infectious Diseases. 2000;**181**:437-440

[33] Taylor-Robinson D, Thomas BJ, Goldin R. *Chlamydia pneumoniae* in infrequently examined blood vessels. Journal of Clinical Pathology. 2002;**55**:218-220

[34] Di Pietro M, Filardo S, De Santis F, Mastromarino P, Sessa R. *Chlamydia pneumoniae* and oxidative stress in cardiovascular disease: State of the art and prevention strategies. International Journal of Molecular Sciences. 2015;**16**(1):724-735. DOI: 10.3390/ijms16010724

[35] Kalayoglu M, Libby P, Byrne GI. *Chlamydia pneumoniae* as an emerging risk factor in cardiovascular disease. JAMA. 2002;**288**:274-231

[36] Grayston JT, Campbell LA, Kuo CC. A new respiratory tract pathogen: *Chlamydia pneumoniae* strain TWAR. The Journal of Infectious Diseases. 1990;**161**:618-625

[37] Paldanius M, Bloigu A, Leinonen M. Measurement of *chlamydia pneumoniae*-specific immunoglobulin a (IgA) antibodies by the microimmunofluorescent (MIF) method: Comparison of seven fluorescein-labelled anti-human IgA conjugates in an in-house MIF test using one commercial MIF and one enzyme immunoassay kit. Clinical and Diagnostic Laboratory Immunology. 2003;**10**:8-12

[38] Ekman MR, Leinonen M, Syrjala H. Evaluation of serological methods in the diagnosis of chlamydia pneumoniae pneumonia during an epidemic in Finland. European Journal of Clinical Microbiology & Infectious Diseases. 1993;**12**:756-760

[39] Schumacher A, Lerkerod B, Seljeflot I. *Chlamydia pneumoniae* serology: Importance of methodology in patients with coronary heart disease and healthy individuals. Journal of Clinical Microbiology. 2001;**39**:1859-1864

[40] Grayston JT. Infections caused by *chlamydia pneumoniae* strain TWAR. Clinical Infectious Diseases. 1992;**15**:757-761

[41] Grayston JT. Background and current knowledge of *chlamydia pneumoniae* and atherosclerosis. The Journal of Infectious Diseases. 2000;**181**:402-410

[42] Saikku P, Leinonen M, Tenkanen L. Chronic *chlamydia pneumoniae* infection as a risk factor for coronary heart disease in the Helsinki heart study. Annals of Internal Medicine. 1992;**116**:273-278

[43] Dowell S, Peeling R, Boman J. Standardizing chlamydia pneumoniae assays: Recommendations from the centers for disease control and prevention (USA) and the laboratory centre for disease control (Canada). Clinical Infectious Diseases. 2001;**33**:492-503

[44] Murray LJ, O'Reilly DPJ, Ong GML. Chlamydia pneumoniae antibodies are associated with an atherogenic lipid profile. Heart. 1999;**81**:239-244

[45] Laurila A, Bloigu A, Näyhä S. *Chlamydia pneumoniae* antibodies and serum lipids in Finnish men: Cross sectional study. BMJ. 1997;**314**:1456-1457

[46] Marangoni A, Fiorino E, Gilardi F. *Chlamydia pneumoniae* acute liver infection affects hepatic cholesterol and triglyceride metabolism in mice. Atherosclerosis. 2015;**241**:471-479

[47] Kalayoglu MV, Byrne GI. Induction of macrophage foam cell formation by *chlamydia pneumoniae*. The Journal of Infectious Diseases. 1998;**177**:725-729

[48] Kalayoglu MV, Hoerneman B, LaVerda D. Cellular oxidation of low-density lipoprotein by *Chlamydiae pneumoniae*. The Journal of Infectious Diseases. 1999;**180**:780-790

[49] Kälvegren H, Bylin H, Leanderson P. *Chlamydia pneumoniae* induces nitric oxide synthase and lipoxygenase-dependent production of reactive oxygen species in platelets. Effects on oxidation of low-density lipoproteins. Thrombosis and Haemostasis. 2005;**94**:327-335

[50] Kol A, Bourcier T, Lichtman AH. Chlamydial and human heat shock protein 60s activate human vascular endothelium, smooth muscle cells and macrophages. Journal of Clinical Investigation. 1999;**103**:571-557

[51] Rosenberger K, Dembny P, Derkow K. Intrathecal heat shock protein 60 mediates neurodegeneration and demyelination in the CNS through a TLR4- and MyD88-dependent pathway. Molecular Neurodegeneration. 2015;**10**:5

[52] Lehnardt S, Schott E, Trimbuch T. A vicious cycle involving release of heat shock protein 60 from injured cells and activation of toll-like receptor 4 mediates neurodegeneration in the CNS. The Journal of Neuroscience. 2008;**28**:2320-2331

[53] Prabhakar S, Kurien E, Gupta RS. Heat shock protein immunoreactivity in CSF: Correlation with oligoclonal banding and demyelinating disease. Neurology. 1994;**44**:1644-1618

[54] Halcox JPJ, Roy C, Tubach F. C-reactive protein levels in patients at cardiovascular risk: EURIKA study. BMC Cardiovascular Disorders. 2014;**14**:25

[55] Rovainen M, Viik-Kajander M, Palosuo MD. Infections, inflammation, and the risk of coronary heart disease. Circulation. 2000;**101**:252-257

[56] Johnston SC, Messina LM, Browner WS. C-reactive protein levels and viable *chlamydia pneumoniae* in carotid artery atherosclerosis. Stroke. 2001;**32**:2748-2752

[57] Johnston SC, Zhang H, Messina LM. *Chlamydia pneumoniae* burden in carotid arteries is associated with upregulation of plaque interleukin-6 and elevated C-reactive protein in serum. Arteriosclerosis, Thrombosis, and Vascular Biology. 2005;**25**:2648-2653

[58] Haubitz M, Brunkhorst R. C- reactive protein and chronic *Chlamydophila pneumoniae* infection—Long term predictors for cardiovascular disease and survival in patients on peritoneal dialysis. Nephrology, Dialysis, Transplantation. 2001;**16**:809-815

[59] Mosorin M, Juvonen J, Biancari F. Use of doxycycline to decrease the growth rate of abdominal aortic aneurysms: A randomized double-blind, placebo-controlled pilot study. Journal of Vascular Surgery. 2001;**34**:606-610

[60] World Health Organization. C-reactive protein concentrations as a marker of inflammation or infection for interpreting biomarkers of micronutrient status. In: Vitamin and Mineral Nutrition Information System. 2014. Available from: http://apps.who.int/iris/bitstream/10665/133708/1/WHO_NMH_NHD_EPG_14.7_eng.pdf?ua=1. [Accessed 25 April 2018]

[61] Jackson LA, Campbell LA, Schmidt RA. Specificity of detection of *C pneumoniae* in cardiovascular atheroma. Evaluation of the innocent bystander hypothesis. The American Journal of Pathology. 1997;**150**:1785-1790

[62] Abdulkarim AS, Petrovic LM, Kim WR. Primary biliary cirrhosis: An infectious disease caused by *chlamydia pneumoniae*? Journal of Hepatology. 2003;**40**:380-384

[63] Yildiz H, Wieërs G, Yombi JC. Liver granulomatosis: A case of *Chlamydophila pneumoniae* infection. Acta Clinica Belgica. 2014;**70**:50-52

[64] Marangoni A, Donati M, Cavrini F. *Chlamydia pneumoniae* replicates in Kupffer cells in mouse model of liver infection. World Journal of Gastroenterology. 2006;**12**:6453-6457

[65] Richardson A, Hawkins S, Shadabi F. Enhanced laboratory diagnosis of human *chlamydia pneumoniae* infection through pattern recognition derived from pathology database analysis. In: Chetty M, Ahmad S, Ngom A, Teng SW, editors. Third IAPR International Conference on Pattern Recognition in Bioinformatics, Melbourne Australia. Berlin, Heidelberg: Springer-Verlag; 2008. pp. 227-234

[66] Skaar EP. The battle for iron between bacterial pathogens and their vertebrate hosts. PLoS Pathogens. 2010;**6**:e1000949

[67] Al-Younes HM, Rudel T, Brinkman V. Low iron availability modulates the course of *Chlamydophila pneumoniae* infection. Cellular Microbiology. 2001;**3**:427-437

[68] Ganz T, Nemeth E. Iron homeostasis in host defence and inflammation. Nature Reviews. Immunology. 2015;**15**:500-510

[69] Edvinsson M, Frisk P, Boman K. *Chlamydophila pneumoniae* changes iron homeostasis in infected tissues. International Journal of Medical Microbiology. 2008;**298**:635-644

[70] Edvinsson M, Tallkvist J, Nyström-Rosander C. Iron homeostasis in tissues is affected during persistent *chlamydia pneumoniae* infection in mice. BioMed Research International. 2017;**2017**:3642301

[71] Ouellette SP, Byrne GI. *Chlamydia pneumoniae*: Prospects and predictions for an emerging pathogen. In: Friedman H, Yamamoto Y, Bendinelli M, editors. Chlamydia pneumoniae: Infection and Disease. New York: Kluwer Academic/ Plenum Publishers; 2004. pp. 1-9

[72] Contini C, Seraceni S, Cultrera R Chlamydophila pneumoniae infection and its role in neurological disorders. Interdisciplinary Perspectives on Infectious Diseases 2010;**2010**:273573. DOI: 10.1155/2010/273573

[73] Gieffers J, Rupp J, Gebert A. First-choice antibiotics at subinhibitory concentrations induce persistence of Chlamydophila pneumoniae. Antimicrobial Agents and Chemotherapy. 2004;**48**:1402-1405

[74] Stratton CW, Wheldon DB. Antimicrobial treatment of multiple sclerosis. Infection. 2007;**35**:383-385

[75] Gieffers J, Fullgraf H, Jahn J. *Chlamydia pneumoniae* infection in circulating human monocytes is refractory to antibiotic treatment. Circulation. 2001;**103**:51-56

[76] Blasi f, Tarsia P, Jackson LA, Grayston MD. Chlamydophila (Chlamydia) pneumoniae—Infectious Disease and Antimicrobial Agents. 2021. (antimicrobe.org/m02.asp)

[77] Mitchell WM, Stratton CW. Diagnosis and management of infection caused by chlamydia. United States Patent, US 6,884,784, 2005

[78] Villareal C, Whittum-Hudson JA, Hudson AP. Persistent Chlamydiae and chronic arthritis. Arthritis Research. 2002;**4**:5-9

[79] Peeling RW. Laboratory diagnosis of chlamydia pneumoniae infections. Canadian Journal of Infectious Diseases. 1995;**6**(4):198-203. DOI: 10.1155/1995/696950

[80] Erkkilä L, Jauhiainen M, Laitinen K, et al. Effect of simvastatin, an established lipid-lowering drug, on pulmonary chlamydia pneumoniae infection in mice. Antimicrobial Agents and Chemotherapy. 2005;**49**(9):3959-3962. DOI: 10.1128/AAC.49.9.3959-3962.2005

[81] Dechend R, Gieffers J, Dietz R, Joerres A, Rupp J, Luft FC, et al. Hydroxymethylglutaryl coenzyme a reductase inhibition reduces chlamydia pneumoniae-induced cell interaction and activation. Circulation. 2003;**108**(3):261-265. DOI: 10.1161/01.CIR.0000083367.93022.78

[82] Koppen LM, Whitaker A, Rosene A, Beckett RD. Efficacy of berberine alone and in combination for the treatment of hyperlipidemia: A systematic review. Journal of Evidence-Based Integrative Medicine. 2017;**22**(4):956-968. DOI: 10.1177/2156587216687695

[83] Kong W, Wei J, Abidi P, Lin M, Inaba S, Li C, et al. Berberine is a novel cholesterol-lowering drug working through a unique mechanism distinct from statins. Nature Medicine. Dec 2004;**10**(12):1344-1351. DOI: 10.1038/nm1135

[84] Kong WJ, Wei J, Zuo ZY, Wang YM, Song DQ, You XF, et al. Combination of simvastatin with berberine improves the lipid-lowering efficacy. Metabolism. 2008 Aug;**57**(8):1029-1037. DOI: 10.1016/j.metabol.2008.01.037

[85] Ma L, Zhang L, Wang B, Wei J, Liu J, Zhang L. Berberine inhibits chlamydia pneumoniae infection-induced vascular smooth muscle cell migration through downregulating MMP3 and MMP9 via PI3K. European Journal of Pharmacology. 1 1515;**755**:102-109. DOI: 10.1016/j.ejphar.2015.02.039

[86] Di Pietro M, de Santis F, Schiavoni G, Filardo S, Sessa R. Resveratrol in *chlamydia pneumoniae* induced foam cell formation and interleukin-17A sythesis. Journal of Biological Regulators and Homeostatic Agents. 2013;**27**:509-518

[87] Deby-Dupont G, Mouithys-Mickalad A, Serteyn D, Lamy M, Deby C. Resveratrol and curcumin reduce the respiratory burst of chlamydia-primed THP-1 cells. Biochemical and Biophysical Research Communications. 2005;**333**:21-27

[88] Rizzo A, Carratelli CR, Losacco A, Iovene MR. Antimicrobial effect of natural polyphenols with or without antibiotics on chlamydia pneumoniae infection in vitro. Microbial Drug Resistance. Feb 2014;**20**(1):1-10. DOI: 10.1089/mdr.2013.0024

[89] Shen ML, Lipsky JJ, Naylor S. Role of disulfiram in the in vitro inhibition of rat liver mitochondrial aldehyde dehydrogenase. Biochemical Pharmacology. 2000;**60**:947-953 https://doi.org/10.1016/S0006-2952(00)00435-4

[90] Johansson B. A review of the pharmacokinetics and pharmacodynamics of disulfiram and its metabolites. Acta Psychiatrica Scandinavica. Supplementum. 1992;**369**:15-26

[91] Long TE. 2017. Repurposing thiram and disulfiram as antibacterial agents for multidrug-resistant Staphylococcus aureus infections. Antimicrobial Agents

and Chemotherapy 61:e00898-e00817. https://doi.org/10.1128/AAC .00898-17

[92] Gao J, Gong Z, Montesano D, Glazer E, Liegner K. "Repurposing" disulfiram in the treatment of lyme disease and babesiosis: retrospective review of first 3 years' experience in one medical practice. Antibiotics. 2020; **9**(12):868. DOI: 10.3390/antibiotics9120868